Pr

"Andrea Leigh Rogers cuts to the chase with her practical tips, clever hacks, and personal stories that will get you unstuck and moving toward the life you dream of."

—Barbara Corcoran, founder of The Corcoran Group and shark on ABC's *Shark Tank*

"*Small Moves, Big Life* is the guide every ambitious woman needs to create space for herself in a world that constantly demands more. Andrea Leigh Rogers offers a refreshingly practical path to clarity, confidence, and energy."

—Aishwarya Iyer, founder and CEO of Brightland

"Endlessly encouraging, truly uplifting, and not afraid to tell you some real at home truths: reading this book is like having a glass of wine with a best friend who really believes in you!"

—Elisa Marshall, founder and chief brand officer of Maman

"Andrea Leigh Rogers has created a must-read for every woman juggling career, motherhood, and self-care. *Small Moves, Big Life* is a game-changer—offering practical, science-backed habits that help us show up as our strongest, most radiant selves. As a mother and entrepreneur, I know firsthand how powerful these small shifts can be."

—Nicole Trunfio, founder of Bumpsuit

"Andrea Leigh Rogers gets it—life is loud, messy, and overwhelming, and women are expected to hold it all together while smiling. *Small Moves, Big Life* isn't just advice—it's a lifeline. Think of it as your daily pep talk from a wise friend with killer abs."

—Jo Piazza, author of *The Sicilian Inheritance* and host of *Under the Influence*

"*Small Moves, Big Life* is a reminder that transformation doesn't have to be overwhelming to be powerful. Andrea Leigh Rogers breaks it down into simple, approachable steps that feel achievable. In a world that constantly pulls us in a million directions, this book gives you permission to slow down, show up for yourself, and build the life you deserve, one small change at a time."

—Brittany Lo, founder and CEO of Beia Beauty

"The motivation any working mom needs to believe that all things are possible with good intention and a positive, driven routine. I will definitely be incorporating these tips into my daily routine. I have been Andrea-fied and I'm loving it!"

—Sharina Gutierrez, *Sports Illustrated* model and founder of Mama Mantra

"These seven simple steps have completely transformed my mornings and my mindset. From the first deep inhale to the final wind-down, each practice is easy to follow, surprisingly effective, and backed by science. I feel more energized, focused, and confident every single day. If you're looking for a way to start strong and feel amazing, this is it!"

—Keni Silva, media personality, philanthropist, and author of *Divorce as an Opportunity*

"*Small Moves, Big Life* is the rare book that's both inspiring and actionable. As a founder, I know how easy it is to lose yourself in the hustle. Andrea reminds us that reclaiming your energy and confidence doesn't require a total life overhaul . . . just a few intentional shifts."

—Natalie Mackey, founder of Winky Lux

"As a leader in the health insurance industry, I've seen too many times what a lack of self-care can do to someone and in many cases, it makes them uninsurable. Through Andrea Leigh Rogers's authentic passion for helping others, she has created seven daily practices that are simple, tactical solutions anyone and everyone should incorporate into their every day."

—Mara Dorne, senior regional sales leader at US Health Advisors

"Running a business, raising a family, trying not to drink myself to sleep . . . life these days can be challenging. Andrea gets it. This book is full of simple shifts that make a big difference."

—Leila Shams, founder, designer, and CEO of TA3 as seen on *Shark Tank*

"Andrea Leigh Rogers exudes joy and light in all that she does, and this book is her good energy personified. *Small Moves, Big Life* is the perfect guide to help all of us pivot toward positivity and overall balance."

—Ashley Bellman, Emmy Award–winning entertainment reporter

"*Small Moves, Big Life* is like a reset button for the modern woman. Andrea Leigh Rogers delivers bite-sized strategies that make a real impact. As a mom, businesswoman, and someone who lives by her calendar, I found this book to be equal parts empowering and practical. Andrea reminds us that taking care of ourselves doesn't have to be one more thing on the to-do list—it can be the thing that makes everything else possible."

—Kirsten Jordan, luxury real estate advisor and national housing expert

"I loved working with Andrea! She always has the most positive attitude and understands how women balance it all. She reminds me to take moments for myself amidst life's chaos!"

—Martha Hunt, former client and Victoria's Secret model

"Empowering, thoughtful, and inspiring, this book delivers relatable advice, real-life strategies, and personal stories to help you unlock your potential and be the person you've always dreamed of becoming."

—Liz Elting, founder and CEO of the Elizabeth Elting Foundation and *Wall Street Journal* bestselling author of *Dream Big and Win*

"An uber encouraging book to help you to start a SIMPLE routine with BIG implications! The book you didn't know you needed."

—Jessica Hart, international supermodel and entrepreneur

"*Small Moves, Big Life* is a breath of fresh air in a world that demands so much of women. Andrea reminds us that taking care of ourselves doesn't have to mean overhauling everything—it can start with one powerful, intentional step."

—Maria Hatzistefanis, founder and CEO of The Rodial Group

"I met Andrea in an elevator five years ago and that thirty-second ride is something I'll never forget. Andrea's energy, passion for health, and purposeful balance are all characteristics that separate her from the pack. I am so happy to see her mantras memorialized for all of us to learn from and to commit to our everyday. Kudos to you, Andrea; this is such an amazing read!!"

—Rita V. Linkner, MD, FAAD, DABOM, board-certified dermatologist and founder of RVLSkincare

# small moves, big life

### 7 DAILY PRACTICES TO SUPERCHARGE YOUR ENERGY, PRODUCTIVITY, AND HAPPINESS (IN JUST MINUTES A DAY)

## andrea leigh rogers

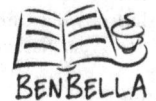

BenBella Books, Inc.
Dallas, TX

This book is for informational purposes only. It is not intended to serve as a substitute for professional medical advice. The author and publisher specifically disclaim any and all liability arising directly or indirectly from the use of any information contained in this book. A health care professional should be consulted regarding your specific medical situation. Any product mentioned in this book does not imply endorsement of that product by the author or publisher.

*Small Moves, Big Life* copyright © 2025 by Andrea Leigh Rogers

All rights reserved. Except in the case of brief quotations embodied in critical articles or reviews, no part of this book may be used or reproduced, stored, transmitted, or used in any manner whatsoever, including for training artificial intelligence (AI) technologies or for automated text and data mining, without prior written permission from the publisher.

BenBella Books, Inc.
8080 N. Central Expressway
Suite 1700
Dallas, TX 75206
benbellabooks.com
Send feedback to feedback@benbellabooks.com

*BenBella* is a federally registered trademark.

Printed in the United States of America
10 9 8 7 6 5 4 3 2 1

Library of Congress Control Number: 2025013956
ISBN 9781637747452 (trade paperback)
ISBN 9781637747469 (electronic)

Editing by Leah Wilson, Stephanie Gorton, and Claire Schulz
Copyediting by Elizabeth Degenhard
Proofreading by Jill Kramer and Marissa Wold Uhrina
Text design and composition by PerfecType, Nashville, TN
Cover design by Kara Klontz
Printed by Lake Book Manufacturing

Special discounts for bulk sales are available. Please contact bulkorders@benbellabooks.com.

*To Leigh and Laine: You are my everything, and I'm so proud and grateful to be your momma. Keep seeing the extraordinary in the ordinary. And to all the women ready to take the next step: This is for you.*

# contents

| | | |
|---|---|---|
| **foreword** | | xi |
| **introduction** | | xv |
| **daily practice #1:** | Breathe In | 1 |
| **daily practice #2:** | Stretch Yourself | 33 |
| **daily practice #3:** | Just Press Play | 61 |
| **daily practice #4:** | Do The Thing | 93 |
| **daily practice #5:** | Set the Table | 123 |
| **daily practice #6:** | Mind Up | 151 |
| **daily practice #7:** | Breathe It Out | 179 |
| **conclusion:** We're on the Trail Together | | 209 |
| **cheat sheet** | | 216 |
| **acknowledgments** | | 220 |

# foreword

## FOREWORD

We all start from somewhere. When I was a young woman, modeling helped me realize my passion for travel, and I found myself en route for Paris soon after high school graduation. It was hard work, but those years spent far from home were truly formative, full of chance connections and new experiences and ideas that helped shape my life—but isn't travel always like that? You never know what will happen.

Later on, when I became a mother, I was living abroad, and despite love from family and friends, the person I had to rely on the most was myself. I knew—above all else—I wanted independence. I had dreams of starting my own business, but it's hard to make your dreams a reality. You know what your heart desires, but you have to figure out how to get there. We don't always have the tools or the understanding to know how to achieve what we really want. Although this is especially true when we are young, it can happen at any age.

That's why I was so drawn to Andrea Leigh Rogers's *Small Moves, Big Life*. It's a smart set of answers to all these questions and—ultimately—an encouraging guide to life. Follow her series of tiny daily actions and, over time, you will find they add up to something truly impressive. These are the tools to help give you the momentum you might need.

I also feel a personal connection to *Small Moves, Big Life*. Like me, Andrea also knows what it's like to be a mom, to run your own global business, and how to balance your own success with the needs of your family. Her story of overcoming her own

## FOREWORD

personal challenges, exceeding expectations, and how her small daily moves help her dig deep enough to achieve all she has is so inspiring.

Reading Andrea's book, I realized I already have a couple of my own Small Moves—and you might feel the same. For me, I draw strength and happiness from spending time with my family. In the last few years, I have used that strength to continue building my own fashion and accessories businesses, and although it's a tough grind at times, it's incredibly rewarding. This independence is so important, particularly for women, and I get there through scheduling and prioritizing, something Andrea is also a fan of. I particularly love her "Do The Thing" chapter, which is a refreshing, foolproof way to truly achieve all you need to.

No matter who you are, what you're doing, or what career you have, you will face challenges (we all do). But you have to believe in yourself. You have to be there for yourself. You have to be strong for yourself—whatever that means for you. And you have to trust yourself. We all start from somewhere, but as Andrea writes, it's really just a series of small moves, with a lot of effort and little self-belief, that will lead you to your Big Life.

—*Dee Ocleppo Hilfiger*
*Fashion designer and entrepreneur*

**introduction**

## INTRODUCTION

First, a little real talk.

Before we begin, I need you to know something important: you don't need to take three months off to eat, pray, and love yourself into a whole new human being (although wouldn't that be fabulous?). You don't need to travel to a tropical five-star health resort—by private jet, natch—to have your chakras expensively realigned. And you don't need to burn half your wages on one of those gourmet meal delivery detoxes. (Hot tip: just eat whole foods and your body will do the work for you.) We're not here to cross our fingers or charge our crystals in the hopes we might magically manifest a dream job, a perfect partner, or a perkier butt. And I don't expect you to start yourself again, from scratch—nobody has time for that.

But if you want things to finally change, for your life to become unstuck, and for your energy, productivity, and happiness to be restored, girl, you're in the right place. Because I have a way forward.

Wherever you are in your life right now, you will have your own reason for picking up this book. Maybe you're in a rut or you're a woman on the verge, or perhaps you have a sense of longing that's growing more and more urgent as time passes. You want to do something more with your life but, somehow, you're not. And yet, your day is full of tasks and responsibilities. This is especially true for those who care for others, bandaging scrapes, fixing school lunches, and coordinating everyone's

## INTRODUCTION

appointments. Although it's rewarding, it's repetitive, and sometimes your life just doesn't feel quite like your own. Weren't *you* supposed to be the main character?

Maybe things haven't turned out the way you'd hoped; something completely out of your control might have happened, or a series of unfortunate events and missed opportunities, and now you're playing an endless game of catch-up. Perhaps you're caught in a feedback loop of scrolling and anxiety, and even though you're busy every hour of every day, your hopes and dreams remain unfulfilled. You want to feel stronger, sleep better, strengthen your emotional resilience, feel like your life has momentum, and also feel great naked (and why not?).

Tradition tells us, as women, that just about everyone and everything takes precedence over our own needs and desires. While we can push against that idea and make sure our kids and the young people in our lives see us doing so, it's a powerful message. Even now, reading this book, the idea of taking a little time—just thirty minutes a day—to center yourself through a series of simple Daily Practices might make you feel a little uncomfortable. You might even feel guilty. *What about my kids? My partner? The housework (and that never-ending pile of laundry)?* Living like this, with your needs constantly coming last, and feeling uneasy when you do anything just for you, can leave you frustrated, unproductive, unhappy, and—let's face it—just completely over it.

INTRODUCTION

# How to Get Your Life Back

We're going to start real small. Just like me.

Growing up, my mom always told me, "Good things come in small packages." To this day, I barely graze the five-foot marker (although I definitely hit it on my tippy toes), but that phrase is something I have held in my heart since I was a young girl. Back then, it showed me anything was possible. "You can do big things, Andrea," I would remind myself. "Just take it one small step at a time."

Slowly but surely, those small steps started to add up. I saw that with consistency and a little effort over time, I could achieve big things.

It all began, of course, with high drama, petty rivalries, and leg warmers. I'm talking kids' and teen dance competitions across the Midwest in the 1990s. Remember that kid at school with the high ponytail, endless sequins and sparkles, headphones glued on, and CD Discman whirring? That was me! But I was tough—tiny and tough—and I learned the steps, put in the hours (so, so many hours), applied a ton of hairspray, and won competitions—lots.

Later, those same small steps secured me a coveted spot as a professional dancer for Disney, my dream job at the time. Afterward, I put in countless hours of study and teaching experience to become a fitness and wellness instructor. Later still, those same small moves helped me grow a little entrepreneurial

## INTRODUCTION

confidence: I fell in love with Pilates and created the Xtend Barre method, opened fitness studios all around the world, became a super trainer online, and—for more than fifteen years—I've been a motivational leader to thousands of women. Oh, and now I'm a mom myself! Did everything go my way? Nope. Was it easy? Not at all. But each small step got me closer to where I needed to be.

Small moves, big life: that's how I've achieved all the good stuff, and when things came crashing down, that's also how I stayed strong and resilient. A few years ago, when I hit that low point—and it was a *really low* point—I found I already had the tools I needed to pick myself up and rebuild a life even better than before.

I'll share more about this low point—and my slow but steady rise out of it—a little later, but it left me in a state of shock. I was in a jewelry exchange parking lot when it finally caught up with me. I sat in my car, holding two watches and my wedding ring in my hand.

Weeks earlier, everything I had been so sure of, everything I had worked so hard for, and all my hopes and dreams and emotional down payments suddenly became null and void. I was now in the last place I thought I'd ever be. My marriage was in crisis, a huge question mark now hung over my finances, and I had two little girls to take care of.

Of course, looking back, there were tiny hints of what was to come. Sure, my husband and I had our issues, but I was in

## INTRODUCTION

love! With a little effort, there was a golden future on the horizon, I was sure of it. But then, life took an unexpected turn, which is the polite way to put it. At the time, the phrase flashing in my mind like a neon sign was more like: "Andrea! Wake up! Shit is literally hitting the fan!"

In front of me, framed by the windshield, was my destination: Boca Raton's classiest pawnshop. It specialized in fine jewelry and watches, and I really needed the money. I had been put in an awful financial position and, although I came into it unknowingly, there I was anyway, in a Boca shopping plaza, about to sell my most valuable possessions.

My whole body was numb. *How am I here?* I wondered, *I've done everything right! How am I in this position?* I'd arranged to meet one of my best friends, the endlessly patient and supportive Desiree, and with her by my side I successfully sold my things and recouped enough money to resolve the immediate emergency. It was truly humbling. I remember walking back out onto that parking lot in the bright Boca sunshine feeling dazed and confused. *How the hell did I get here?*

The tools I used to eventually rise up, discovered through trial, error, and instinct, were integral to pulling me out of the gloom and into the light—and keeping me there. They became a series of Daily Practices, and even now, I do them without fail, seven days a week.

There are 7 Daily Practices in all, and each one is rooted in science. They felt right from the very beginning (and that's

## INTRODUCTION

usually enough for me), but I researched the heck out of them. Knowing each one has stats and studies behind it, for me, really gives them an edge. We'll start and end with breath—something you're already doing right now—with stretching, a mini-workout, and more in between.

Each section of this book contains instructions for both your basic practice and next-level practice. But even if you only do the minimum—and that's where I started—you'll still see incredible results.

Done throughout the day, but mainly in the morning, and adding up to *just thirty minutes in total*, consistently doing these 7 Daily Practices has incredible transformative power for your body and mind. In fact, I challenge you not to fall in love with how far these small moves will take you.

But right now, you're deciding whether to commit, so you need to know the essentials:

They don't take long.

They're pretty simple.

They will improve your physical and mental health, give structure to your daily life, and make you feel great. Hopeful, even.

Oh, and they'll improve your motivation, too.

Maybe you'll still book that eat, pray, love tropical five-star chakra realignment trip instead (let me know how that goes!), but if you're looking for a realistic route and a trail partner who can give a lot of friendly encouragement and a little tough talk now and again, I got you.

INTRODUCTION

This was my way forward: a series of small steps to get me permanently out of the rut and onto the good stuff. It really, really works, and it could be your way, too.

## Navigating the Rut

So, why are so many of us stuck in that rut in the first place? Why are women so often desperate for more energy, to achieve more, and to have more to look forward to? Short of ringing an alarm bell, some of us aren't in a great place. Online, at work, at home—in every area of our lives—as women, we're expected to do it all and have it all. No wonder we can feel burnt out sometimes. That kind of pressure leaves us feeling stressed, discouraged, and increasingly exhausted, both physically and mentally.

Pulled in every direction, so many of the women I meet professionally and personally tell me they're just not able to use their time in a way that is effective or particularly fulfilling. They struggle just to maintain the status quo, never mind make space for change, and they fall a little short of the confidence and sense of achievement that's essential to happiness.

Many of us feel bad spending any amount of time on self-care and renewal. From childhood to our teens and our college years with all the pressures of studying and socializing, to our first jobs and first serious relationships, we can lose sight of ourselves. Becoming a mom also has its challenges, and the level of selflessness it demands can be overwhelming. There is even

## INTRODUCTION

a name for this feeling: "mom guilt," which we'll get into later. As psychologist Sherrie Bourg Carter says, many women "see themselves as the one[s] who should be taking care of everyone else, and their needs often fall by the wayside." Some of us are really trying hard, achieving little, feeling crappy and guilty, and can't see a way out.

We'll explore a little science surrounding habit formation later in this book, but—put simply—objects in motion stay in motion. And objects that are still, well, they stay that way. This is the power of the rut: once you're in it, you're in it. You're the stationary object, and no matter how much you want the opposite to be true, hoping and wishing will not aid your escape. The longer you're in it, you'll probably start to feel worse, your motivation will flatline, and you'll feel crappier and guiltier than ever. The rut has claimed you.

Unless you do something about it. Here's what I know to be true: a series of small Daily Practices, done consistently with each one completed in a few minutes, will help you navigate your way out of the rut for good.

## Finding Your Voice

The most wonderful women I know often cannot think of a single good thing to say about themselves! For the past few years, I've run a series of retreats in the United States and Europe. We mix a little culture, cuisine, and exploration together with a lot

## INTRODUCTION

of movement, and some really delicious wine. I love the immersive nature of a retreat. It's an intense way to learn, but I find that all of us are more receptive and open-minded when we're in an unfamiliar but beautiful environment, away from our everyday selves. Although incredibly rewarding, hosting a retreat can be a challenge, so I love to over-prepare, and I like to think I'm ready for anything. Still, every single time, there is something that surprises me.

With that in mind, I need to tell you about a retreat I hosted a couple years ago in Beaver Creek, Colorado. The hotel, which overlooked beautiful mountain meadows and the Gore Range, had the most amazing spa and was just drop-dead gorgeous. On day one, right after my welcome address, I was excited to try a new warm-up exercise I'd created. There were about thirty women there, and I knew it would be a surefire way to quickly break the ice and create instant connection between all the guests (I consider a retreat a success if my attendees all swap numbers at the end; it gives me the feels!). I especially love that first morning when everyone's wide-eyed, a little nervous, a little out of their comfort zone, but excited for what's to come.

"I want everybody to think about a person they love," I said. "It could be your best friend, your mom, your spouse, whomever; just think about the person you love; really visualize them . . ." I soon saw a smile start to spread across the faces of everyone in the room; it turns out it's impossible to think about someone you love without smiling.

INTRODUCTION

"Now, I want you to walk around the room and shout out—really shout out—all the things you love about them, as loud as you can!" I remember a few surprised looks, but within moments the bravest attendee shouted: "Kindness!" and then another voice said, "Her laugh!"; it set everyone off, just as I'd hoped. They were shouting and marching around, and I was encouraging them, giving them my best Disney shout-outs: "I can't hear you! Keep it going!" It got loud, and fast; the volume cranked up to eleven, and even I was surprised—I hoped the hotel had prepared themselves for the roar of thirty happy women. At the end of that part of the exercise, we were all flushed, laughing at having done something potentially embarrassing, but with the undeniable support of everyone else in the room. But they didn't know my plan; I wasn't done yet.

We all took a moment, sat down, caught our breath, and talked a little. Then I got them moving once more. "Let's do that again, get those legs moving, that's right . . ." They thought they were ready this time, excited to go another round of something that was now familiar—but they were wrong: "Let's change focus," I said. "Now we're going to shout out everything that we love about . . . ourselves!" I remember each attendee looking up at me, mystified. "Go!" I said, excited to hear the roar again. But not a word was spoken. It was dead silent.

I knew it would be a challenging task for relative strangers to share something positive about themselves, but even I was shocked at how these women who were shouting out loud just moments before now stood quiet and still. This was a group of confident, successful women, some of whom had flown halfway around the world for this retreat. And they couldn't think of a single positive thing to say about themselves.

It was eye-opening for all of us. I'm happy to say we eventually uncovered many positive personal discoveries during our time together, but it made me wonder: Why are we so down on ourselves and our own potential?

In our discussions, we explored the idea that we're taught, as women and girls, to both limit our successes and how we communicate them. While women have made huge strides in the world, many of us are still unable to release our attachment to older gender roles, and that attachment defines how we view our own potential. We can do *good* things, but not *great* things. Just like we're only allowed to do girl things, not boy things. We can be the senior executive but don't expect to make CEO; the nurse, not the surgeon. We're wary of intimidating others—men—and setting off their insecurities. So we find ourselves tempering our achievements, imposing limits on our desires and interests, doing everything for everyone else, and we lose our voice and sense of self in the process.

Even the wonderful women on my retreat, each one of them truly accomplished, found it uncomfortable to share their successes. But sharing our triumphs might just inspire others, helping us all rise above the very gendered expectation to live a little life. Why can't we easily name something good about ourselves, and why can't we proudly shout it from the rooftops?

INTRODUCTION

## How We'll Do it

Over the next seven sections, we'll work on escaping the rut and finding that voice by going deep into each Daily Practice. You'll learn exactly how to do each one, try out a few different versions, and then decide on which one works best for you. That way you can personalize the whole system.

Remember, there are just seven things to do, and some take just a couple of minutes to achieve. You'll be surprised by how simple and effective they are and how confident you'll feel from the outset. Plus, you'll get to know a little of the science behind each one, so you'll know for sure this is all heading somewhere good.

I'll also include a way to level up each Daily Practice so that, once you've mastered each one, you can go even further (although if you just stick to the basic method, that's great, too!).

We'll get there via personal stories and realizations, and you'll also meet some of my personal heroes, incredible women who've really been there and lived to tell the tale, and who can shed their own unique light on their favorite practice.

First up, we'll take a deep inhale and try out some morning breathing exercises to find an invigorating clarity, slowly wake the body, and fix a determined mindset for the day ahead. Second, we'll discover the benefits of conscientious stretching techniques followed by the third step, a targeted and full-out ten-minute mini workout (that's the sweaty part, but it will be over before you know it, and it will make you feel amazing).

Fourth, we'll discover an unbeatable rethink to the classic to-do list; fifth, a breakfast self-care rule that will change the way you think about food; sixth, an easy verbal practice of self-love; and finally, for the seventh and last practice, we'll exhale together via a no-excuses restorative wind-down for successful sleep.

Got all that? Now, maybe it's a little early in *Small Moves, Big Life* to be so honest, but I promised a little real talk, right?

None of this is rocket science.

In fact, this whole system is pretty simple. Your jaw will drop when you see how easy—and how effective—day one is going to be. These are very small moves, and it will feel absolutely in your power to achieve every single one of them. But think like you're training for a teen dance competition in the 1990s: little steps add up.

Stick to the *Small Moves, Big Life* program—really, really stick to it—and you'll develop energy you never knew you had, rise above feelings of worry and self-doubt to become more resilient and upbeat, and find the motivation and commitment to meet all your everyday objectives—and maybe even have the mental space to fulfill your most ambitious hopes and dreams.

## Why It Works

These practices are daily for a reason. Once you've put in the time—remember, just thirty minutes total every day—they'll become habits, and, over time, your new habits will do the

## INTRODUCTION

heavy lifting for you. In a 2021 study published in the *British Journal of Health Psychology*, researchers built upon the theory that habits are formed through a three-step process: cue, routine, and reward.

This process, they showed, becomes automatic over time. Do a thing at the same time and same place every day, and eventually it will stick, helping you achieve a reward (in this case, feeling badass).

So, developing an everyday ritual—and revisiting the same time and space in which you do that ritual—matters a lot to healthy habit formation. It doesn't happen overnight but, as some daily practices take just two or three minutes, embedding a ritual will come sooner and easier than you think.

Some of you will pull this off in a matter of weeks (well done, you!), while for others it will take longer. But I can promise you right now, if it takes a little more time than you'd like for your 7 Daily Practices to become habits, you won't care at all—because you'll start to feel the benefit of them immediately.

Once that healthy habit is hardwired, your mind will be able to refocus on even more high-value activities. Your short-term challenges dealt with, you can turn your attention to long-term dreams. You'll have a stronger foundation, and you'll really feel it: that increased energy and a sense of calmness when things hit the fan.

You'll also have more mental space to focus on your long-term goals, whatever they are. Former president Barack Obama once told reporters, "You'll see I wear only gray or blue suits. I'm trying to pare down my decisions. I don't want to make decisions about what I'm eating or wearing. Because I have too many other decisions to make." Simplicity and consistency are paramount.

## Now, Let's Do The Thing

Working with women, hearing their stories, and seeing their untapped potential—from incredible strength to a capacity for love, success, and happiness—has truly inspired me. I wrote this book for both the young woman who is heading off to college and the mom who is dropping her off. I wrote it for first jobbers through to CEOs, long-term caregivers and full-time moms, and my best friend, Risa, who is forty-seven, single, successful, and endlessly curious about living that next phase of her life with purpose.

And I wrote it for you.

All of us are unique, and what works for some women won't work for everyone. But when it comes down to it, so many of our challenges are the same—haven't we all broken down in a parking lot, in a manner of speaking?

When I felt my knees buckle (emotionally and literally), I looked for something tiny I knew I could accomplish. I pulled together a morning routine of small, focused tasks to shift my attitude and make me feel capable and strong again. The simple act of doing something productive every day—and repeating

## INTRODUCTION

it—gave me the foundation of confidence I needed. These are my 7 Daily Practices, developed through science and personal experience. They lifted me up, and, from there, my way forward was to acknowledge a deep desire to do something I felt proud of. I wanted to have a positive impact on the world and the women around me, and—whoa—I knew I needed to do something to make me smile again. So, after many years, here it is: *Small Moves, Big Life.*

Let this book sit on your nightstand, within arm's reach, pages folded and highlighted, phrases underlined; whatever gets you there. But mostly, let yourself hold one amazing possibility in your mind: very, very good things are ahead.

You just need to make your move.

—— **daily practice #1** ——

# breathe in

*powerful rhythms of inhalation and exhalation
to help you re-center,
no matter what is happening
in your life*

> **WHAT WILL I BE DOING?**
> Simple breathing exercises.
>
> **HOW LONG DOES IT TAKE?**
> 2 minutes, minimum. That's it.
>
> **WHEN DO I DO IT?**
> In the morning, first thing, and as needed throughout the day.
>
> **AND WHAT WILL I ACHIEVE?**
> Improved mental and physical health, emotional resilience, and the secret to everlasting youth (kidding, but only that last part).

Every day,
    every hour,
every minute,
you take a breath.

But how often are you truly aware of your breathing?

I'm talking about a *real* breath. That last breath you took before diving into the ocean, that deep, satisfied exhale at the end of fitness class or a sunset run, or filling your lungs before you take on a power ballad at karaoke. (My go-to is "Total Eclipse of the Heart" by Bonnie Tyler, and it's a quite a sound.) Even blowing out candles on a delicious birthday cake or gently puffing away the powdered sugar from a delicious Italian pastry, our breath powers life.

Breathwork—conscious, mindful breathing—is, I know from experience, the foundation of a positive, motivated, get-things-done outlook. And doing just a little, every single day, has incredible transformative power.

I have tried out some of the world's most time-honored breathing techniques and put them to work. I've explored their incredible and sometimes surprising effects, tracked down the academic research (in short, the more research there is, the more breathwork comes out on top), and made breathwork an integral part of my daily routine; and I've taught hundreds of women how to do the same.

As simple as it may seem, breathwork has been a cornerstone of my career as a professional dancer and Pilates instructor, business owner, leader, and even as a mom. And, as I have seen over and over again among the women I work with, breathwork is the surest way to relax, energize, and focus as you prepare to take on new challenges.

For many years, as a dancer, I used breath instinctively. It fired up my body, cooled and calmed my mind, and helped me survive life's toughest moments. But it wasn't until I studied Pilates and understood the startling science behind breathwork that I realized its true potential, its quiet power as a daily practice, and how—combined with other rituals—it can be a game changer.

At one end of the scale, breathing is involuntary. It's just something we do, a reflex our body will fulfill on its own via our autonomic nervous system. We all know, with a little biology class knowledge, that our body extracts oxygen from each inhale, enough to go about the business of living, and with each exhale, it expels what we don't need in the form of carbon dioxide—and all this happens without us even thinking about it. Breathing oxygenates our bodies, helps fuel energy, and improves our ability to concentrate. At the other end of the scale, well-practiced breathwork can override this involuntary act; we can guide it, harnessing its power to help deal with truly traumatic events, perform incredible physical feats, and even enter trancelike states.

But I'm interested in the sweet spot right in the middle of that scale—where breathing with depth and clarity through simple techniques, performed daily and with real consistency, can support and improve your physical health, and your emotional health, too. Like all my Daily Practices, the health benefits are proven, and just a single session can have a positive effect, but the real trick is doing breathwork each and every day, to create a cumulative effect on your health and mindset.

And so, this is what I know to be true: conscious breathing, done with real awareness—for just a couple of minutes a day, every day—is really, really good for you, from calming your mind to soothing your sympathetic nervous system. There it is. Welcome to Daily Practice #1.

First thing in the morning, every morning, I want you to devote two minutes to basic breathwork.

Over the next pages, I will show you powerful techniques that are science backed (and in one case, Navy SEALS–tested!), and describe which of them can be your go-to solutions for different daily challenges. There is breathwork to energize when you're feeling low, breathwork to calm when you're anxious or irked, breathwork to counteract screen apnea (that zombie-like state caused by too much scrolling), and breathwork to encourage a little sleepiness at the end of the day.

Once you've mastered these techniques, I also want to give you room to go even further, to level up and introduce breathwork whenever you need it throughout the day. For that, I've saved my own signature breathing series to share with you—the one I do every single day, without fail, either before getting my girls ready for school, before the dog walk and matcha-making (I'm weirdly obsessed with matcha; it's almost becoming a problem), in the car pool line, at the checkout, after a tough meeting, and anytime I'm feeling anxious or overwhelmed.

I'll help you discover which technique is best for you, when to work it into your day, how to use it as a powerful tool in a crisis (hopefully few and far between!), and why breathwork is an essential element of my 7 Daily Practices.

Will Daily Practice #1, breathing mindfully for two minutes a day, save your life? No, of course not. But will gradually and consistently managing your stress through small, easy actions like breathing exercises have a positive and measurable effect on your general physical and mental health? Girl, yes!

As you go about crafting your own daily ritual, you can use the specific breathwork pattern that works best for you (or might fit a specific challenge you're having in the moment). I'll introduce you to six options for breath patterns in this chapter.

I almost always do mine in the morning; I'm the first one up in my house, and there is something about that early morning quiet that I love. Most days are crazy, but that quiet moment—before it all begins—is the perfect time to do my Daily Practice #1.

But maybe your perfect moment is different. Perhaps it's in the bathroom as the shower is running, in the elevator at work, or at your home-office desk, just before your first Zoom of the day. Maybe it's waiting in line at the grocery store, just before your class at the gym, or in your car in the parking lot of your favorite Italian bakery (just me?). I don't mind when, so long as you do it.

What's more, I want you to think of Daily Practice #1 as a starting point, a place to grow from. Commit to doing the minimum two minutes without fail, which is the important part, but also keep an eye on taking things to the next level, adding in extra or longer breathwork sessions as you get better and better at it (and I promise you will).

Worried you don't have time for a daily breathing practice? Let's get real: you do, and you can. I know you can. Just devote two minutes to consciously do something you already do every minute of every day anyway.

## BREATHE IN

Up first is belly breathing, designed to energize. It's simple, effective, and a great place to start:

---

### belly breathing

**WHAT IT DOES**
Boosts energy

**TIME IT TAKES**
2 minutes (or more if you're feeling it)

**HOW TO DO IT**
Sit comfortably, place your hands on your chest and stomach, and close your eyes. Breathe in deeply, concentrating the inhalation from your belly, and—with your hands—feel your belly and lungs expand, and count to 5. Then, without holding your breath in between, exhale for another 5 counts—in a relaxed, normal way. Repeat for 2 minutes or more.

---

Feeling energized? Just a little? As I explain how I discovered my other favorite techniques, we'll head to Toronto, South Florida, and across the Caribbean. But first, let's start a little humbly, in the dance studios of the Midwest. Trust me, this will all make sense!

## Breathing with Instinct

From the age of three and throughout my childhood and teens, I performed in countless dance competitions—and I loved every glittery moment of it. I was a tiny mover and shaker. Name a strip mall studio, school gymnasium, or community center in Michigan and beyond, and I have probably danced in it. By the time I was a teenager, I wasn't just performing. I was also a choreographer and had even started teaching the little three-year-olds in my local studio. I just couldn't get enough.

Dancing competitively from a very young age, I had always used the power of breath to move my body—but breathwork wasn't taught, and it wasn't really thought of as a skill. Instead, it was something completely instinctive. Even as a kid, when I took to the stage, I just knew when I had to take that inhale, and when I had the exertion of a big move, I knew I would have to exhale. I had to really use my breath, somehow aware of the power it holds. It not only helped energize my dance moves, but it also helped me concentrate and calm my mind so I could connect with whatever my focus was, like remembering a complicated new routine.

I already knew that if I was just doing the moves and not concentrating on my breath, my mind would go anywhere and everywhere. But when you're a teenager in athletic training, with your mom driving you to dance class five or six times a week, you're not really thinking about these words or concepts,

# BREATHE IN

and you're most definitely, 100 percent not interested in how breath has power. You're thinking about Brandon and Brenda in *Beverly Hills 90210*, Oprah interviewing Michael Jackson on live TV, or when the new Counting Crows album is out (please don't judge—it was the 1990s, and "Mr. Jones" is still one of my favorite songs). You're just doing it.

Or, when you're a kid rushing in from playing rough-and-tumble games in the backyard, barely able to catch your breath, you're not thinking about how air fuels you and how it might also calm you—you're just deep in the moment, leaves in your hair, dirt smudges on your nose, having fun.

Back then, I would do my homework in the hallways of my dance studio, in between classes or grabbing a bite to eat, and I learned how to multitask and balance life. As I grew older, the one thing I craved was a professional dance role, but I knew this wasn't going to be a dream easily realized. No one else in my family performed and, although they completely supported my passion, it seemed to make sense that I continue my academic studies and get a "real" job. I could dance all I liked in my spare time, couldn't I? And, I mean, let's get real: How many people actually have a successful career dancing?

In the end, I went to college, and even though I was focused on my classes, I just couldn't get dancing out of my head. I studied communications and thought I might find a career in broadcasting or marketing, something that would answer the creative need in me. But part of me knew I was just going through the motions. I was doing what was expected, what I was supposed to do, but not what made me feel alive. And, so, I would often find myself reading the audition papers—as one does when you're a dancer, professional or not—daydreaming of the what-ifs and could-bes.

And then, during my summer at home between my freshman and sophomore year, I saw a job posting that changed my life.

A major audition was taking place the very next day, and nineteen-year-old me thought the role was perfect. I had to have it. Disney Cruise Line was contracting a small number of actors, singers, and dancers for a yearlong contract to perform for guests on voyages across the Caribbean. Those who passed the audition were to become part of a theatrical repertory company at sea, traveling the world, and learning and performing several musical shows. It would mean leaving home, leaving college, living on a cruise liner, and becoming part of the Disney family—something that made that little mover and shaker in me spark. But most exciting, it would mean working with the highest caliber of artists and creatives I could imagine— something I had dreamed about for years. It might not have been a starring role on Broadway, or performing at the Folies Bergère in Paris, but for this Midwestern girl, back then, it was all I wanted.

*This is it*, I thought. *This is what I need!*

The catch? The casting call was in Toronto, five and a half hours by car from my home in Michigan. Call time was 8 AM, and I had only just discovered the job ad at around 3 PM that afternoon—there was less than twenty-four hours to go.

I called my mom, who immediately said, "You have to call your father."

So I did. "Dad, I've got to do this," I said.

Without hesitation, he replied, "Alright, I'm coming home."

He left work early, and we packed the car together while my mom booked a hotel in Toronto. I should point out here that my parents are those kind of people: incredibly supportive, endlessly generous with their time and energy, both with a can-do attitude I have tried my best to center in my own life. They would drop anything to help me, and that day they did. But what does all this have to do with breath? We're almost there, I promise.

We drove through the night, arriving at our hotel in the dark, and they delivered me to the audition the next morning—we did it!

But, in those final moments before call time, stretching in the hallway with a long line of talented performers, I suddenly felt it: a wave of anxiety. It was a situation I had been in hundreds of times before, only this time it felt different. I had always worked hard to be good at my craft, knowing it would help me achieve my goals. The competitive dance world was not rocket science to me, and I knew if I gave it my all, I had a chance. But now it felt as though my entire future depended on this moment. My chest grew tight.

It took my breath away.

Doubts started to race through my mind. I had just started college, and now I had taken my parents on—what? A wild-goose chase? To Canada? And there were dozens of others who had worked just as hard as I had to be there. My chest grew even tighter. Could I even do this?

I couldn't catch my breath.

I was about to perform in the biggest audition of my life, and I couldn't breathe. And so, there was nothing to do but force myself to slow down and steady my breathing.

Dance is almost always about the eight count. That count lies underneath every piece of music, every beat, every choreographed move, and it's ingrained in every physical performer like a sixth sense (I can feel my toe tapping out the rhythm as I write this). So, in that hallway I used that magical eight count to guide my breathing. Instinctively, I slowly inhaled to the count of four, then exhaled for four.

Inhale for four, exhale for four.

My body felt like it was fighting me, but I did it again and again, rhythmically syncopating my breath to the dance beat inside my head. And, after a few moments, my chest started to feel looser, more expansive, and my focus slowly returned.

Years later, I discovered I had been doing a variation of breath counting, an ancient technique that is delightfully simple and proven to be effective.

Here's how to do it:

BREATHE IN

## breath counting

**WHAT IT DOES**
Brings calm and focus

**TIME IT TAKES**
2 minutes or more

**HOW TO DO IT**
Breathe in through your nose—as you would normally—and count each breath, in your mind. One inhale and exhale count as one breath. Keep most of your attention on your breath and only a little on your counting; it's okay to be distracted, but if you lose count, start again from 1. Goal is to work up to 10 breaths (10 inhales and exhales).

## The Science of Stress

When you feel stressed, or your emotions are heightened, your sympathetic nervous system, or SNS, fires up and jumps into action. You might have heard it described as a fight-or-flight response; your body makes and releases adrenaline, the stress hormone, at an elevated rate. Your pupils enlarge to improve your vision, blood rushes to your muscles and heart so you can make a quick getaway, you're sweaty and covered in goose bumps, and your physical body energizes and readies itself for action. What's more, your nerves seem to sizzle, you might tremble, and you are breathless with anxiety. In other words, you're at DEFCON 2.

But our bodies often misjudge the threat and react out of proportion to the perceived hazard. What might have once saved our life from prehistoric dangers—giving us the ability to fight for our lives or run like the wind—now switches on at even the mildest snafus of modern living.

Perhaps you have just received a difficult email, the *ding!* of a worrying news alert, or an unexpected phone call (why is that such a jump scare these days?). Your body will ready itself to survive mortal danger, releasing a surge of adrenaline that is, almost always, unnecessary.

When this kind of stress response becomes habitual, it puts an incredible strain on your heart and may additionally drive inflammation, increasing the risks of obesity and other chronic health conditions. But the good news is that lessening your stress response and learning to manage it can genuinely improve your health.

And the science backs all this up. Although I always think of California as the most chill state, in late 2023 a female-led research team from the Salk Institute for Biological Studies in sunny San Diego published a fascinating report on the link between stress and illness. We've long known that stress wears us down, undermining not just our emotional outlook, but our general physical health, too. But the Salk researchers, led by

Professor Susan Kaech, discovered further proof of what many have suspected all along. There is a relationship between noradrenaline (a neurotransmitter released from the sympathetic nervous system, acting as a stress hormone that fires up when you're surprised or scared) and our T cells, those friendly killer cells that are vital for immunity. The noradrenaline clings onto the T cell, zapping it of its energy, and leaving it less effective in fighting off illness. The Salk team found that by lowering or blocking the amount of noradrenaline in the body, T cells were able to spark back into life and do their job. Incredible news, considering that T cells attack cancer cells.

Kaech's team used medication to achieve their results, but it follows that lowering your levels of stress and managing your reaction to stressful situations, however you do it, will improve your health.

That's where breath comes in.

Breathwork activates the parasympathetic nervous system, counteracting the body's well-intentioned but misguided tendency to escalate its stress reflex. By slowing down and taking deep breaths, you can lower your heart rate—whether you simply want to relax or focus, or you are trying to slow down a full-on panic attack. That's exactly what I found myself doing in the moments before the biggest audition of my life.

The audition began. I danced and danced and made it through every callback until the very end. Then I was dismissed with the usual "We'll call you if you get the role."

We drove home to Michigan, exhausted but happy. I had that sense of achievement you get when you know you've done something huge, something full of potential, and I think it was a day or two later when I got the call. It was the casting agent calling to ask if I did en pointe work—the ballet term for dancing on the tips of your toes.

"Oh, yeah . . . sure, of course," I said, making my voice sound cheery and not full of fear. "I absolutely do!"

The truth was, I hadn't done it in years.

"Great," he said. "Can you send me a videotape?"

"Sure I can," I replied, not knowing how I would do any of this, but knowing I had to. I hung up and felt that same feeling again: the anxiety I had experienced right before the audition. And so, again, I slowed my breath, counting as I did it—four counts in, four counts out—until calm was restored.

After my instinctive breathwork had calmed and energized me once more, I searched through the house for my old pointe shoes (please still fit!) and, when I found them, I called my dad once again. I told him I needed to dance on camera and then mail the tape to the casting director in Toronto as quickly as possible. And once again, he took a breath and simply said, "I'm on my way."

I performed my en pointe moves while Dad held the camcorder, and we FedExed the tape overnight. The following afternoon I heard from the casting director: "Andrea, I just want to congratulate you." I remember standing in the kitchen, hearing those words, the phone at my ear, knowing my life was about to change, and for a moment I was speechless. "I just want to congratulate you," he said again. "You got the job." The feeling was electrifying.

"Oh my gosh," I said, finally. "That's amazing! So, you got the video?"

And he said, "Yes, but I didn't even open it." I couldn't believe it. "I didn't need to," he went on. "I already knew you had the talent. But now I know you have diligence. And that's what got you the job."

It was one of my first big life lessons. Not only do you have to work hard enough to shine, but you must also manage your anxieties, be organized, and show up. Oh, and you need a great support team, whether it's family, friends, or your own sense of inner strength.

Years later, as I was studying breathwork and making it a nonnegotiable part of my every day, the memory of my Disney audition came back to me. I remembered how my first, amateur attempt at mindful breathing had truly centered me, allowing me to reach a state of energetic calm so that I was able to truly pursue my dream.

Within weeks, I had paused my college career and was living in Toronto, learning my moves, and about to set sail across the Caribbean and off toward my future. I couldn't wait to get started.

## Remembering How to Breathe

After my year with Disney and my first experience of dancing professionally on the high seas, I found it hard to go back to those college classrooms in Michigan. I felt like I'd pressed play on my life and built real momentum, and now I was forced to press pause.

But the experience had given me real hope, and with years of training in self-discipline and finishing whatever I started, I knew I couldn't quit college. *Andrea, I know this doesn't suit your soul right now*, I said to myself, *but you are just going to have to keep your head down and do this. And you're going to be grateful you've finished.* If I wanted the success and adventure I dreamed of, that I'd already had a taste of, I had to do the thing. So I doubled up on classes; even with my year out with Disney I could still graduate on time.

Years later, I realized the importance of that attitude. If we do the hard thing, bit by bit, our lives start to flow. Today, it is something I talk about with the women I coach. Whether you're doing breathwork, stretching, improving your sleep routine, or just finding time to sit down to eat. Whatever it is you know you need to do, you just need to do the thing. Just do it. And, as I discovered, once you start to become that person who does the thing, it doesn't leave you quickly. Do the thing, and it becomes easier and easier; it self-perpetuates.

But sometimes anxiety can sneak up on you. Feeling nervous and panicked after sitting at your screen for long periods, performing on endless video calls, gossiping on Slack, clicking through shopping sites at sale time, or scrolling endlessly on your phone just seems like modern living. There's a name for it, though: email or screen apnea. Writer Linda Stone wrote about the phenomenon in *The Huffington Post* in 2008 and, well, it resonated. Her anecdotal study (she rounded up two hundred friends, friends of friends, and work colleagues and got them to self-monitor as they checked their emails) seemed to prove her theory: that screen time can, for some reason, unconsciously slow down or even stop our breathing, or make us breathe in a shallow, rapid way. None of these options are good. They can kickstart your sympathetic nervous system, causing that fight-or-flight response. What's more, shallow breathing or holding your breath for long periods of time means your body and brain are not getting the oxygen they need—and the brain, more than anywhere else in the body, needs a lot of it. Shallow breathing can even cause problems with concentration (it's why your mind can go blank in times of stress).

Answering your emails, which is really a list of potential problems and challenges to solve, can put you in a state of nervous anticipation. Science writer James Nestor, whose 2020 book *Breath: The New Science of a Lost Art* is now the go-to for understanding screen apnea, recommends setting up breath reminders—and I would add a posture check and stretch breaks to that, too. Do everything you can to get away from your screen for short periods and make breathing easier with an open and expansive body. In 2023, a study out of Stanford seemed to show that a few minutes of daily breathwork really does improve mood and reduces anxiety caused by things like screen apnea—more than meditation alone. A specific technique came out on top: cyclic sighing. Here's how to do it:

### cyclic sighing

**WHAT IT DOES**
Calms screen-time terrors

**HOW LONG DOES IT TAKE?**
2 to 5 minutes (the Stanford team recommends 5 minutes)

**HOW TO DO IT**
Sit comfortably or lie down. Breathe in through your nose and expand your belly (this will fill your lungs about halfway), then pause for a moment, and then breathe in again, fully expanding your lungs and chest, and then—slowly—exhale in a sigh, for longer than your inhale. Repeat.

## How Breath Powers Movement

After college, I moved to South Florida. I had met a man and fallen in love, and we married and hit the road days after graduation. I had hopes of discovering a fresh take on life, a happy, purpose-driven, more "adult" existence. But I soon realized it didn't matter if I was in snow boots in Michigan or living by the sea in South Florida: I had this incredible drive but nowhere to put my energy.

I knew I needed to go back to what made me feel alive, what made me spark. After a period of floundering, I realized that movement was my passion. It's what filled my lungs with hope and made me feel like I was floating above the clouds—and it's always been that way. I had left my dance and movement community behind me, but without something like dance in my life I was never going to find my purpose. I needed to move.

I found I had a natural affinity for Pilates, and it soon became an essential part of my training and conditioning; it made me strong, kept me supple, and protected me from injury. It even made me feel a little closer to one of my own contemporary dance idols, Paula Abdul, who loves my studio brand, Xtend Barre (but more on that later). And in South Florida, I discovered Pilates as a career. I soon found myself enrolled in a classic comprehensive Pilates course, studying anatomy and physiology, learning the classical Pilates moves and how each one flows perfectly into the next. As I discovered the core principles of Pilates, I once again learned that our health and happiness are powered by just one thing:

Breath.

I remember reading that in my textbook late one night and having a light-bulb moment: "Oh my gosh, I already know this. I've been doing this for years." And I hadn't even realized it.

In those Pilates classes, when I inhaled purposefully through the nose and exhaled deep from my core, known as lateral breathing, every class, for weeks on end, I really started to feel it: *Wow*, I would think, *I'm so present in this move, I'm so here right now. And it feels so great, like I've been up a mountain on a retreat for three months.* My breath was connecting me to the present, to the here and now. It was powerful.

I thought back to that Disney audition, and an idea jumped into my mind: I could make conscious breathing a habit. Breath started to become the solution in situations where my stress levels were heightened. I would remember how I'd felt in class, how calm and in-the-moment I had been, and I would go back to my Pilates principles. With that in mind, another breathing technique I love is what I call "expansive breathing," which is an alternative to belly breathing (page 7). Often when you are stressed or anxious, you will feel it in your chest; everything is tight, and it feels like you are not getting enough oxygen. Or—by way of analogy—you might think of what it is like to wear skinny jeans and eat a serious dinner. When you get home, it is the most amazing (and necessary) relief to take off those constricting pants. You feel instantly relaxed and liberated—physically and emotionally!

BREATHE IN

## expansive breathing

**WHAT IT DOES**
Busts stress and grounds you

**HOW LONG DOES IT TAKE**
2 minutes

**HOW TO DO IT**
Sit or lie down comfortably, one hand on your chest, one on your belly, and check your body for tension, relaxing your shoulders. Slowly inhale through your nose, filling your lungs, and breathing into your back ribs and expanding from left to right. With each inhale, imagine your whole trunk expanding further and bringing with it a liberating energy and lightness.

## Breathing When It All Hits the Fan

It wasn't until I went through a life-changing experience, years after that Disney audition, that using breath outside of the exercise realm became essential. From my earliest days as a Pilates instructor, I gained a loyal community of (mainly) women who loved my classes as much as I loved teaching them. From there, slowly and painstakingly, I built up my own fitness empire, an evolution of the system I called Xtend Barre, with dance, Pilates, barre work, and great music. (I haven't yet found a way to add

Counting Crows to the playlist, but I will!) It is fun and sweaty, and I'm so proud of it, and it's now delivered in a series of studios around the world. When my career started to pick up speed, I found myself trying to keep up with my international expansion. Even though I am very driven, a dedicated student, and a big dreamer, at that point in my life, speed-learning the intricacies of big business was a challenge.

I also had two amazing, very young girls at home and, as a relatively new mom, I was desperate to be with them as much as I could. Soon, I was stretched too thin. I had "mom guilt," and for the first time in my life, my love for movement and Pilates, my yearning to grow a business for my family, and my determination to be there for my kids were truly tested.

And then, for me at least, the world suddenly stopped spinning.

After seven years, in 2013, it was all uprooted: my husband and I were about to end our marriage.

We had a wonderful life, and a wonderful future, all mapped out. We had two children. We were in love. And now, suddenly, he wasn't sure he could continue. It looked like it was over. I was in complete shock. How could this be my life?

I was completely numb and, not for the first time in my life, I couldn't catch my breath.

Somehow, I made it through the dark days that followed, but the feeling of fear and dread soon caught up with me. I was shopping for groceries in Whole Foods, walking slowly along the aisles with my shopping cart, in a daze, and I suddenly felt it, a wave of emotion crashing, my knees buckling underneath me. *Oh my God*, I thought, *I'm going to collapse. I need to hold on to this cart just to stay upright.* Somehow, step by step, I carried on walking through the store, picking up groceries, paying at the checkout. Incredibly, I was still smiling at people—I didn't know what else to do—but inside, I felt like I was dying.

I still couldn't catch my breath.

I got home and just sat there, inhaling and exhaling, clutching the smudge spray I'd just bought in the store, hoping it would cleanse and calm me, just like the label claimed. I would spray it into the air—it seemed like such a hollow, harebrained thing to do in that moment, but I would have tried just about anything—and I focused on my breathing, on its rhythm and depth.

*You got this, Andrea*, I told myself, although I wasn't sure I believed it.

Perhaps I was craving the structure I'd had as a child? All those training programs and performing in competitions had left me with little time to sit and worry, but maybe I'd also had too little time to contemplate life. I found myself returning to breath again and again. It took weeks, but somehow I got to the point where I needed to do it a little less and less every day.

Slowly, I was able to reclaim my breath.

Ultimately, breathwork brought me back to a more positive mindset. My perspective started to shift; I stopped feeling like a negative blob and started to pull myself out of that trainwreck way of thinking.

I was a young woman with two young babies and a man I cared about very much, so I was determined to save my marriage. In the weeks and months that followed, I tried to make things work. I let breathwork power me, and each tiny step I made gave me a little more confidence, a little more belief in myself. But the more I believed in myself, the more clearly I could see that I was trying to fix the unfixable.

Of course, many of us have experienced this kind of heart-stopping panic, and things much, much worse than a marriage ending, but there is a commonality to these big crises. To the body, sudden grief, the shock of illness, losing your job, and divorce are all the same. When something completely unexpected and awful happens, it's an emotional gut punch, and a literal one, too.

It will surprise precisely no one to learn that women are disproportionately affected by stress. The American Psychological Association has long tracked the "gender gap" in how much stress American men and women self-report, and their findings are consistent: women are more likely than men to be chronically stressed and anxious.

I know breathwork can help. Eventually, I turned to a technique favored by Navy SEALS, box breathing, as my calming, anxiety-combating practice. There's a reason why box breathing is the go-to for Navy SEALS to calm and control their stress response. It's an effective, easy-to-learn skill that can be done

BREATHE IN

almost anywhere at any time, and it can be a tool for you in the most difficult times of your life. Here's how it's done:

---

## box breathing

**WHAT IT DOES**
Calms in impossible, tough-ass situations

**TIME IT TAKES**
2 minutes

**HOW TO DO IT**
Start by exhaling all the air from your lungs, and then pause to the count of 4. Inhale through your nose for 4 counts, hold your breath for 4 counts, and then exhale steadily through your nose for 4 counts. Importantly, try to keep an expansive, open posture as you exhale (it's tempting to curl in on yourself), and repeat the process several times.

---

The SEALS will do this for several minutes, working their way up to ten or even twenty minutes as they start to see the benefits of daily practice. They need it: being in the military is, of course, one of the most stressful jobs there is. Box breathing—so-called because of its four equal steps—will help you clear your head and zero in on what's important. This technique is a wonderful example of controlled breathing.

As I inhaled and exhaled like a Navy SEAL, I told myself, *You got this*, only this time I also gave myself a little dancer's advice, too, something I'd always murmured to myself before I took stage: "Chin up, toes pointed." It means you're ready to move.

*Chin up, toes pointed, Andrea: go.*

Breathwork helped steady me, powering my slow but satisfying transformation toward confidence and self-belief. I soon incorporated breathwork into my daily practice and did it consistently, without fail. Four years after the first crisis in my marriage—and four years stronger—I could see that the life I was trying so desperately to save wasn't the best thing for my future and wasn't the best thing for my family. Slowly, little by little, I had grown and, finally, I had the courage to let go.

I told myself: *Girl, you've got so much ahead. You are meant for great things. You are meant to live an incredible life. And you are going to continue to raise these wonderful children and meet a wonderful man.*

## Now It's Your Turn

From using breath instinctively as a dancer, to understanding the true power of breathwork while studying and practicing Pilates and using it to transform my mindset in a time of acute stress, I finally discovered the importance of breathwork in everyday life.

Today, I find myself coming back to breathwork constantly. When I'm in the carpool line and lacking patience, I think about my breath. If I'm nauseous, I think about my breath. For sustaining energy, for calming, and for clarity—there are just so many different situations where breath is my go-to—it's almost become like a security blanket, the same as that blankie or little stuffed animal you hold on to when you're a kid, the thing that lends comfort and control.

When I talk to the women in my life, through my role as a coach, educator, or just as a friend at the bar over wine (a delicious glass of Sancerre, please), I often hear stories of how we lack the level of comfort and control that we crave. At times, we can feel overwhelmed with the everyday tasks of life; it's like we're treading water—or slowly sinking—and breath can be a tool that keeps us buoyant, keeps us lifted, and keeps our heads above the water.

I turned to breath at a horrible time in my life, but then a beautiful thing happened: slowly, and through consistent, daily practice, I bloomed and blossomed. I became the strong woman I knew I could be, and breath continued to hold me up, and still does, each and every day. With this in mind, a few years ago I developed my own breathwork practice I call Inhale and Xtend.

## How to Level Up Your Breathwork

The point of any breathing exercise is to release tension throughout your body, and, combined with a long exhale, the effect is truly calming. The power of a long exhale is backed up by science. When trying to deactivate or slow down your SNS fight-or-flight response through breathwork, researchers measure your heart rate variability (HRV). HRV is the variation of time between heartbeats and turns out to be a great way to measure general health and fitness. Noticing how our HRV briefly increases as we inhale but decreases as we exhale, researchers discovered that doing the latter stimulates your vagus nerve to secrete a little acetylcholine, a natural substance that slows down your HRV. Put simply, extending your exhale for a few more beats for at least two minutes stimulates the nerve, which ultimately lowers your heart rate variation: like a built-in, all-natural chill pill.

This final signature breathing series has become my "drink of choice," and it's detailed step-by-step below. This technique has helped me to find my breath again and to embrace life with joy, reverence, and confidence.

## inhale and xtend

### WHAT IT DOES
Allows you to pause and focus

### TIME IT TAKES
2 minutes

### HOW TO DO IT
Inhale deeply for 4 counts, slowly extending your arms above your head as you breathe in. Then,

BREATHE IN

hold your arms above your head, stretching your spine long, and hold your breath—for 4 counts. Finally, exhale for 8 counts, extending your arms on either side of your body as you bring them down toward your waist. As you do so, open your chest upward and feel your spine lengthen and gently stretch.

---

I do this every morning, usually when the house is at its most quiet, the girls are still asleep, and our dog, Chedi, is sleeping and quietly snuffling in his crate. I'll sit cross-legged in bed or stand bedside with my feet hip distance apart. With each of my four repetitions, I feel myself waking up; I feel gratitude; I feel relaxed and confident in my body; I feel like I am taking control of my day—and who doesn't want that?

And that's it.

That's what Daily Practice #1 is.

Just two minutes of audition-winning, divorce-surviving breathwork that's science-backed, ancient knowledge–inspired, and proven to improve your physical and mental health.

Try each one—belly breathing, breath counting, cyclic sighing, the Navy SEALS box breathing, or my own Inhale and Xtend variation—and discover which one suits you best. You decide.

Allow yourself some space to level up and add breathwork whenever you need it throughout the day. But, right now, all I want from you is a commitment of just two minutes.

It will be done before you even finish thinking about it. Write a reminder on a sticky note and stick it to your bathroom mirror, the coffee machine, the back of the front door, anywhere you know you'll see it, and just do the thing.

Breathe in. Each and every day.

## daily practice #2

# stretch yourself

*a startlingly simple stretch routine to wake up your body, restore your energy, and sharpen your mind*

> **WHAT WILL I BE DOING?**
> Mindful stretching. You know, like the warm-up we always skip before our workouts.
>
> **HOW LONG WILL IT TAKE?**
> 3 minutes, minimum.
>
> **WHEN DO I DO IT?**
> Each and every morning, right after morning breathwork.
>
> **AND WHAT WILL I ACHIEVE?**
> Stretching will wake up your body, restore your energy, improve your posture, and underline the connection between your mind and your physical self. Stiffness and creakiness will ebb away, muscles will feel elongated, and it can even improve your mental clarity and lift your mood.

Okay, let's stretch.

Right after morning breathwork, nothing wakes up my body more easily and happily than three minutes of gentle, yoga-inspired stretching. Within just a few moments, it simply makes me feel good. You can do it seated, standing, walking, or in bed, if that's where you need to start. If you stretch while still under the covers, number one, you're going to feel better when you get out of bed. And number two, you've already gotten a little movement in for the day. You're also going to be a little more inclined to move your body in a more focused, challenging way, maybe even with a short exercise routine—but more on that later.

Why do it? There are profound, all-encompassing, and surprising physiological benefits to gentle stretching. Besides making you feel more limber and less creaky and stiff, stretching can ease back pain, help with sleep, prevent injuries and headaches, improve your posture, and slow down or soothe chronic illness—there's a reason stretching is a core component to physio and rehab. Oh, and there is evidence it can prolong your life, too.

So that's what we'll be doing here: mastering simple stretch routines, learning about their incredible physical and mental benefits, and incorporating your favorite stretches into your own 7 Daily Practices. We'll learn the basic moves—each powerful in and of itself—add in some mantras to have in mind as you're doing them, and explore how to take it to the next level (via a trip to Japan).

But first, there's something else I need to share with you.

Stretching, like breathwork, has a powerful side effect.

And that side effect is its surprising connection to meditation.

A simple stretch routine, done consistently each and every day, not only increases flexibility and a sense of physical ease and preps your body to work efficiently, but it has also been shown to produce chilled-out, Zen retreat–style mental effects similar to deep meditation. Ask any yoga fan and they'll agree.

Stretching can reduce anxiety and increase a feeling of vitality by releasing serotonin, boosting oxygen levels, and improving blood flow, and create a sense of inner calm. It combines unique physiological effects with all the key benefits of meditation—with minimum effort!

I've performed a morning stretch routine for years, and I know firsthand how transformative this low-effort, minimal-time practice is. As a dancer, stretching before movement sessions is integral, but as a person preparing for the day, whatever it holds, it feels just as important: you don't have to be a dancer, Pilates lover, or yoga expert to be a good stretcher. And, for me, discovering the link between stretching and meditation was a game changer.

To truly incorporate stretching into my own 7 Daily Practices, I researched the science backing up its benefits, discovered what happens to the body during periods of inactivity and how stretching truly wakes us up, and put some of these ideas to the test in Japan, where I made an incredible discovery in terms of stretching and moving to access meditative states. I also learned how to stop scolding myself for doing it imperfectly and how to take pleasure in going my own way (it's okay to get it wrong sometimes!).

Just before we begin, I need to remind anyone who's nervous that this stretch routine is truly gentle. The goal here isn't landing your splits, or crashing down dramatically to the ground, one leg extended in a drag-queen dip (unless that's your thing—in which case, wow); it's about feeling mobile and healthy. It's about gently warming up your body and taking a moment to connect to your physicality, and ultimately having a body that withstands injury and feels good to live in. All this through a little stretch routine every day? Yes. Gentle stretching is winning.

There are lots of kinds of stretches—dynamic, ballistic, passive, and active—and your ultimate Daily Practice will see you holding poses, or making small movements, while counting to ensure every part of your body gets the same attention. We'll explore each kind together, discover one to avoid, and I'll then ask you to implement your favorite in your own morning practice. Allow yourself space to grow; once you've mastered the basic moves, consider going a little further, exploring slightly longer routines. But, right now, all I'm asking for is the minimum. Do you have three minutes every morning to stretch? Of course you do.

From Pilates to yoga and beyond, I've truly tried every stretch going, but I find dynamic stretching to be the most effective and mindful for me. I get to move through any discomfort as I am counting off my repetitions and focus my mind while I do it. The opposite is static stretching, which means positions are held comfortably and completely still through your counts, often at the end of a workout.

Can you overstretch? Well, yes. But we won't be doing that here. Expect to feel a little tightness and tension, but stretching shouldn't be too challenging and definitely not painful in any way. Ballistic stretching, once a fitness industry favorite, is now frowned on as a potential injury-causer. The idea was to push your body into a series of overextensions, stretching beyond your normal range of motion. You would get deep into a position, and at the limit of how far your body could stretch, bounce even farther. Ballistic stretching is now thought to potentially damage the body and even tighten the muscles you are trying to elongate. Again, that's why gentle stretching is best.

Passive stretching is usually aided by a prop like a band, leaning against a wall, or even with an exercise partner, all of which can help intensify your stretch while you simply lie there like a wet noodle and relax. Active stretching is similar but without the props or gym buddy to help; you maintain the stretch with your own muscles.

No matter what stretching practice works best for you, you can reach every part of the body and reap amazing benefits.

So, for Daily Practice #2, I just want you to stretch gently, mindfully, and with consistency to wake up your body and connect you to it. That's all.

Let's get right to it with the forward focus, the gentlest stretch in this repertoire:

## forward focus

### WHAT IT DOES
Awakens the body and gently activates
the abs and upper body

### TIME IT TAKES
2 to 3 minutes, minimum

### HOW TO DO IT

1. Lying on your back, slowly reach both arms to the ceiling and, after gently nodding forward, chin to chest (this helps avoid any strain on your neck), use your abdominals to lift your upper body, slowly lifting your spine off the floor (or bed).
2. Sitting upright, extend your arms toward your toes and relax your neck muscles as you reach forward. Inhale for 8 counts, hold for 2 seconds, and then exhale for 8 counts. Repeat for 2 to 3 minutes.
3. With each inhale, think about the obstacles that lie before you in the day ahead; with each exhale, gently push away the worry.

---

How are you feeling? All stretched out? Not enough? Think you can go a little more? Good.

I know the effectiveness of stretching, and I also know that no matter how busy your morning is (or how raucous your kids are), we can all find three minutes to stretch when we first wake up. You might be raring to get up and start doing the "productive" tasks of your morning. Not so fast! According to recent surveys, the average American spends only about fifteen minutes a day on self-care. The time you take for morning breathwork and stretching—even if it is only five minutes in total—needs to be nonnegotiable.

You need to make it clear to your partner, roommates, family, pup, and most important to yourself, that this is *your* time. Unsurprisingly, this is a special challenge for the parents of young kids, and that is why it is all the more necessary. One Pew Research poll from 2018 found that 74 percent of parents of kids under eighteen reported feeling "too busy to enjoy life" at least part of the time.

Setting aside this time doesn't have to be an exact science. Much like eyeballing my way through recipes when I'm in the kitchen, when it comes to stretching, I like to freestyle my timings. I'm not one for saying, "Alexa, two minutes on the timer," though that works for many. I have that same early morning urge to reach for my phone as most of us, so for me it's better that it's out of the way for a moment. I want to start scrolling and catch up with messages, but I don't, right? Well, not always. I'm not perfect. But I think, *Andrea, get your breathwork done, and your stretching, and then you can do the rest.*

*When* you do your stretch routine is important, however. It's most useful after a period of inactivity, which is why first thing in the morning, right after your two minutes of breathwork (aka Daily Practice #1), will be the most effective time to stretch. If you get up and feel stiffness, aches, or slowness and don't address those sensations, they will chase you throughout the day. They will sneak into your posture and even haunt your mood because you don't realize, until you stretch mindfully, that you might be holding stress and tension in your body.

## Stretch Yourself Awake

Here's something we all share. You can invest in a $10,000 Tempur-Pedic mattress; you can have an ergonomical pillow, premium CBD drops, silk sleep mask, and sleep in the very best body position, but when you first wake up, your body will be stiff and tight. This is true of all adults, regardless of age and health. That slow-to-move, slightly inflexible sensation is common to us all, and not just in your joints but also in your fascia—those layers of membranous connective tissue that support your organs and muscles.

In fact, let's hear it for the fascia. It really doesn't get the love it deserves. It's truly amazing: it really holds everything together, kind of like a mesh bag of oranges, only with a gel-like lubrication between each of its layers. That lubrication, hyaluronic acid, is heat-sensitive, and it gets more slippery and slidey when it's warmed up and with everything in motion. But, because our body temperature generally drops at night, and we're lying still for several hours, everything gets a little stagnant. That lubrication gets thicker and gloopier, the fascia can't slide around as easily, and we feel stiff. It's the same deal for our joints: they are also naturally lubricated but, after a period of inactivity such as sleeping, the cartilage at the ends of our bones drinks up the hyaluronic acid, and we can feel creaky just after waking.

Other considerations are our muscles and our tendons, the incredibly strong tissues that connect our muscles to our bones. Again, through periods of inactivity, our muscles contract a little, they shorten and grow tight, which means that when we try to use them—for exercise, active chores, or just our normal morning movements—they don't extend to their full capacity. This puts extra strain on our joints, muscles, and skeletal system, ultimately putting us at risk of injury, which even a small, sudden movement can trigger.

It can happen to some muscles and not others. For instance, sitting at a desk for hours every day can temporarily tighten your posterior thigh muscles, which means walking or picking something up from the floor will be a little harder. And hunching toward a screen—a monitor or even our phones—will put strain on our necks, shoulders, and upper backs. It's even earned itself a nickname: tech neck. Do this day in, day out, and your lack of flexibility can cause pain. If you've ever hurt your back from something as easy as picking up a sock to put in the hamper, this is probably why. Stretching helps protect against all this. It allows the muscle a practice run toward whatever it is you're about to ask of it, blood flow increases, and those muscle fibers get to elongate.

If you're anything like me, your stretch practice will reveal a few home truths: *I didn't realize I'm so tight*, you'll think, or *I didn't realize I'm holding all this stress from the way I slept last night*. The good news is that, through a daily stretching routine, we can quickly and effectively reawaken our bodies, change the consistency of that lubrication, cut out the creakiness, stretch and condition our muscles and tendons, and set ourselves up for the day ahead, whatever it holds.

With that in mind, let's try the spinal twist, to gently "wring" the tension out of our bodies and activate our muscles, fascia, and joints. It's slightly more challenging and a little more active than the forward focus, and I would suggest doing it on a yoga mat or towel on the floor, or on your bed if it's firm enough.

## spinal twist

### WHAT IT DOES
Awakens the spine, particularly the lower back and abs

### HOW LONG IT TAKES
2 to 3 minutes

### HOW TO DO IT

1. Lie on your back with your knees bent and feet flat on the ground, and extend your arms out to either

side in a T shape, lying them flat on the ground, palms facing down.

Gently raise both knees, bringing them in toward your chest—this is your starting position.
2. Then, lower your knees to the left, letting them slowly drop to the floor together. Your knees should be stacked on top of each other, and your shoulders gently pressed down with equal pressure. Look toward your right hand. You should feel a subtle stretch in your lower back, hips, upper back, and shoulders.
3. Inhale/exhale for 8 counts, and focus on the opposition between the right and left sides of your body; think your way from your tailbone up to the crown of your head, from your right hip across to your left.
4. When you're ready, lift your knees back up and drop them on the opposite side, and repeat.
5. Add a pillow or two for support where you need it (for example, under your knees).

---

If you're a yoga fan, you'll notice that this is similar to the supine spinal twist, or Supta Matsyendrasana. Like all classic yoga moves, it has ancient roots; yoga is thought to be around five thousand years old, but the type adopted by the West, the one that seems to be practiced in almost every American neighborhood, has its own contemporary twist. There's a focus on posture, stamina, balance, and whole-body fitness through stretching and holding different positions. Even though I'm a Pilates girl through and through, that gets a yes from me.

## STRETCH YOURSELF

Follow Adriene Mishler, aka Yoga with Adriene, online (if you're not already). Her free yoga content is an ideal gateway into the art. Her perfectly honed classes are delivered from a simple sunlit studio complete with her dog, Benji, who pads in and out of view. With her calming, friendly, and down-to-earth vibe, it's hard to believe she's one of the most followed yoga teachers in the world (almost 13 million of us subscribe to her YouTube channel). Allow yourself to be inspired by Adriene's moves, and perhaps borrow some of her simple stretches for your own Daily Practice.

Some of us are chronically inflexible—not just because of a long sleep or late-night desk-work session, but as the result of long-term inactivity. Perhaps we're recovering from an injury or illness, or we've just lost motivation and it's easier to sit life out for a beat (trust me, I've been there). My strong belief here is that, however old we are, we're just too young for that. Way too young. But just as we can become less flexible incrementally, we can reverse this process incrementally, too, through gentle stretching. Perhaps it might take a little longer as we age, but you'll get there. (If you have an injury like a strained muscle, the gentler the better. Talk to a physician, physical therapist, or personal trainer to find ways to stretch that help your injury heal rather than aggravating it.)

So, how did I come to use stretching as one of my daily essential practices? Again, it started with dancing. In training, we had to stretch to achieve each position, and if we wanted to compete at the highest levels, those positions had to be perfect. In my head, dancing is 90 percent active stretching, all the time. You call on your body's flexibility and mobility to do crazy tricks, leaps, and turns, and you can't do any of it with just strength. And while it's a great idea to develop your musculature—especially in your later years—it's just as important to stretch your way toward mobility. Stretching also protects you from injury, the dancer and athlete's nightmare, when even a small, temporary injury can put your career back.

I did something a little off-brand recently and found myself engrossed in a football playoff game. I was in awe of the balance, strength, and flexibility exhibited by the players. When one player went for the ball, he suddenly looked so graceful, like a dancer. I started talking at the TV, as you do: "Get the ball . . . get the ball!" And I watched in amazement as the player leapt for the ball, reaching high at the same time, both legs out. "He just did a *grande jeté* for that ball," I said (that's the classic ballet move in which you leap with both legs straight, one behind, one forward). His legs weren't quite straight, but he had huge hip length and reach, and he caught the ball with ease—and the crowd went wild. "Oh, he's got a good mobility coach," I said, nodding to myself, as if I were the new house expert in football. But he could not have caught that ball by just being strong. He also needed the mobility and flexibility. It got me excited, thinking how stretching can help you achieve the greatest things. I think I became a football fan in that moment!

It's not just dancers and athletes who need to hear this. We should all work toward being strong and flexible in equal parts. Now, don't you want that for your personality, too? You want to be strong, to hold your own, but not be so stubborn that you stay stuck in the same spot and never move, right? Flexibility in your physical self—and in your wider life—allows you to evolve and move through life more easily.

An even more active stretch is the hip and heart opener. It's a powerful stretch that uses gravity and body weight to stretch out your hips and back, especially if you're a desk-dweller. Be mindful of your lower back here and only fold forward without feeling uncomfortable—even if it's only an inch or two.

## hip and heart opener

### WHAT IT DOES
Focuses on your hips and back

### HOW LONG IT TAKES
2 to 3 minutes.

### HOW TO DO IT

1. Sit on the edge of your bed with equal weight distribution on your sit bones. Cross your right ankle across your left thigh, opening your hip and keeping your knee and hip in horizontal alignment, if possible. You might be able to do this unaided, but it's okay to use your hands to gently lift and guide your leg into this position.

2. Concentrating on your posture—firm and upright with a long back—slowly lean forward over your right leg, leading with your heart as you flex and fold your hips. You should feel a stretch in your hips, but be mindful to only go so far—as little as an inch or so if that's what you need.
3. Inhale for 8 counts, exhale for 8 counts. As you count off your breaths, affirm the ways you will lead with your heart today. Repeat with your left ankle across your right thigh.

## Stretching for Your Life

In the West, at least, we live in a culture in which looking good has social value. Open Instagram and you'll see an endless grid of "perfect" bodies. It follows that improving how we look is the main reason many of us work out. To put it simply, most of us want a perky ass—and why not? It's not a crime, and if that's your main motivator, well, good for you.

But in terms of our fitness goals, things have started to shift a little—and I think this is a very, very good thing. I see it in my Xtend Barre studios, and I hear it on my coaching calls: we work out not just because we want to look sexy, but we also want longevity, health, and to feel good mentally. Although I want a great derriere, too, I also want to be able to pick something up off the floor when I'm seventy-five.

Flexibility in your later years is a great goal to set your sights on. This is something well understood in the Blue Zones, those tiny geographic areas where communities are generally healthier, residents have fewer chronic diseases, and people simply live longer. There are countless theories as to why these groups seem to thrive, but they all eat healthfully, are sociable, and move and stretch—lots.

In the early 2000s, following a paper published in the journal *Experimental Gerontology* about Sardinian life expectancy, National Geographic Fellow Dan Buettner drew attention to these groups when he came up with a system of Blue Zone locations. He had spent the late 1990s exploring the world, performing record-breaking cycling feats, and he became fascinated by the health of the different communities he passed through. From the shepherds of Sardinia, Italy, to the gardeners of Okinawa, Japan: How was it that they seemed to live longer than others?

With the help of National Geographic, Buettner helped kickstart decades of longevity research into the Blue Zoners and founded an industry of life guides, diets, and exercise programs designed to make use of the Zoners' knowledge. He noted—among other things—how low-intensity activities dominate their days. In these Zones, moving and stretching every twenty minutes or so adds years onto the average lifespan, so it makes sense that these communities include lots of wonderful older people living their best, most flexible lives—even without pickleball. Some are even skilled in the deep squat, giving them incredible hip mobility. They don't fall as much, their cores are stronger, and they have a closer connection with their bodies. Oh, and there's something else Blue Zoners have in common: many of them enjoy a glass of wine now and again. That's something I can get behind.

And it's not just the Blue Zoners who are ahead here. Every time a new sports science paper is published, or new stretch research is revealed, the link between stretching, longevity, and general health is underlined. One of my favorite stretch studies is the legendary National Health Interview Survey, a groundbreaking, long-term project tracking the health habits of more than twenty-five thousand Americans, spanning almost seventy years so far. It started in 1957, and every fifteen to twenty years or so, researchers publish a wealth of data. Of course, the more active participants are, the longer they live, but the study found that stretching was "uniquely associated with lower risks of mortality" (as was volleyball—go figure!).

Since the early days of Buettner's project, not all the original Blue Zones seem to still qualify; sedentary modern living has taken over. But the learning here still holds true: the more mobile you are, every day, the longer you live. And it all starts with a stretch.

## Stretching Mantras

If you're only interested in the physical benefits of stretching, that's fine; they're incredible on their own. But a next-level aim—one I want you to achieve while reading this book and trying out each Practice—is to improve and maintain your mental health, too.

By now, you've tried at least one stretch routine (if you haven't, go back and try one now—it only takes three minutes). And you've not only improved your physicality; you've also accidentally meditated. That's right—whether you knew it or not—you've spent some time becoming aware of your body and actively focusing your mind.

Yep, you've Zen-ed yourself, just a little.

It follows that your stretch routine (and your breathwork practice) can also be an opportunity to throw in some positive thinking. Whether I am doing a morning stretch or an awareness walk (more on that below), I always like to ground myself with reassuring mantras.

Here are just a few of the mantras I love:

**Gratitude Attitude:** I approach every task and every challenge with thankfulness.
**Extraordinary Ordinary:** I put on "extraordinary" glasses for the day and see that even ordinary things can be magical.
**Purpose and Passion:** I live up to my purpose and let my passion fuel my goals.
**#mindup and #heartup:** I #mindup by turning my energy and thoughts to the positive. I #heartup by being kind,

taking a breath, and trusting myself. I know what's best for me. (If you follow me on social media, you know all about #mindup and #heartup already. If not, click on through!)

For me, a person who finds it hard to be still for more than a few moments, the idea that stretching can be a kind of meditation session is a delightful one. I know intimately how powerful meditation can be, but for years I have found it a challenge to consistently add it to my daily life. I'm a mom, I run my own business, and, before I truly implemented my 7 Daily Practices, I sometimes struggled to keep up with myself. Sitting still seemed impossible.

## How to Stretch Yourself Further

It took a change of mindset, a journey to the birthplace of Japanese Zen, and more than a little mental flexibility for me to meet my meditation goals. But I now know that focusing on stretching and slow, soft movement can also help take care of the mind.

I put some of these ideas to the test in Kyoto, Japan, where I made an incredible discovery linking stretching and meditative states (and learned how to stop scolding myself when I couldn't quite keep it up perfectly).

Traditional meditation never worked for me. Guided or solo, for three minutes or thirty, in a circle of crystals and candles, even with a dreamcatcher wafting in the breeze, I just couldn't get there. What's more, I'd get anxious. I know that's the whole point of mastering meditation, but, dammit, I'm a mover. I've been a dancer my entire life, and I rarely sit still. I knew meditation was truly life-changing for many, but I could never find that feeling of calm if I had to keep my body still. And yet, I continued to be fascinated by it.

For this book, in 2024 I traveled to Japan in search of experiences that might further inform my 7 Daily Practices—and scratch that meditation itch I've always had. I have always been drawn to Japanese Zen, especially its focus on awareness and the idea that balance and peace are achieved through training. As a dancer, I had already learned that if you put in the hours, anything is possible. I had hopes of meeting and learning from an expert, a Japanese Zen master who might help me explore my ideas and conquer my resistance to being still. I already knew my own version of zen came when my body was in fluid motion, feeling the rush of energy reaching out to every limb—I'm a dancer, after all. But I was sure there was something I was missing.

First of all, I love Japan. As much as I wanted to try everything, go everywhere, and immerse myself in the country, I wanted to quietly observe, too. From my perspective as an onlooker, a Westerner, and a woman from Midwestern America, I was wowed by the art and architecture, the balance between ancient ways and modern technology, and sprawling cities that seemed impossibly clean—I mean, the public toilets look like how I imagine Martha Stewart's bathroom would be. I also loved the cultural focus on respect: toward the food that's on the table, toward others, and toward the shared environment; it's common to take your trash home with you. A friend's husband worked in Tokyo for many years, and every Friday they would all, from the receptionist to the CEO, clean the office, from the desks to the restrooms. Most of all, I love how travel makes us super aware and open to new ideas, and forces us to be flexible in our thoughts and feelings. Japan certainly opened my eyes.

Through my translator, Masakithai, I was connected to Toryo Ito, a Japanese Zen monk in Kyoto who invited me to meditate with him. Although I was excited about our meeting, something about the situation made me a little nervous. I wanted to approach our session with profound respect, but the idea of being physically motionless for I-don't-know-how-long left me tense, and I started to feel a little of that old anxiety I get when I must sit still.

Toryo and I arranged to meet in the grounds of the ancient Ryosoku-in temple in one of the oldest monasteries in the city's Gion district. As I walked slowly through the tea gardens, all rain-fresh and somehow both wild and manicured at the same time, I thought about the weight of those hundreds, even thousands, of years of history behind the practice, and I felt tiny in comparison.

I thought about the reality of living in the modern world, and my own restless place in it. Could something so ancient, something that seemed so formal, and something that required such stillness really inform and improve my life?

I walked up the temple steps and took my place, cross-legged on the creaky wooden boards of the large veranda looking out onto the lush greenery and lizard tail plants crowned with white leaves. The wider temple complex dates to 1358 but has only been open to non-monks interested in zazen Buddhism since 2018 and, when Toryo sat down opposite me in his dark, traditional robes and lit a stick of incense, I honestly felt as though I had traveled back in time. I tried to focus my mind, knowing I might be in for a long ride.

That's when I saw it, a bright flash as it caught the light: Toryo's Apple Watch. Although I kept my surprise a secret, I remember the quiet shock of it in my body, and I started to smile. I thought, *Girl, you got this kind of wrong, didn't you?* I was jolted back to the present, to the here and now. Toryo had an Apple Watch! Well, of course—why the heck wouldn't he? He's a cool modern monk, and ancient ideas can exist alongside new ones—it's how good the idea is that counts.

Toryo then told me what I really needed to hear: that it was okay to not sit entirely still, that swaying or rocking back and forth was perfectly fine to help get deeper into a state of meditation. "Don't chase it," said Toryo. "No perfectionism." I remember feeling so relieved and, oddly, the knowledge that I didn't have to be as still as a statue meant I was probably the most motionless I have been in all my waking life!

After our seated practice, Toryo informed me we would be trying a walking meditation—applying the same concentrated focus to our bodies and surroundings as we walked. I was delighted and surprised to hear this. With this revelation, Toryo affirmed and validated my approach to stretching and its meditative powers.

As I have already said, I find dynamic stretching to be an effective mindfulness practice for me, and for years I have also practiced what I call awareness walking. As I struggled to sit still and meditate like every article, app, and YouTube tutorial had told me is the secret to achieving a little zen, I found my own solution: mindful walking.

This has been even more important to me since the arrival of my dog, Chedi. Although he has his moments, having a young dog has more benefits than cuteness overload. Walking with him in the early morning hours through the light of sunrise, looking at the world through his eyes, taking in the sights and smells, the crisp air—and doing it without fail, every day—truly has had positive mental health effects.

I shared all this with Toryo, and off we set on our walk, zazen-style. He explained the power of staying present when moving, of contemplating every step, and focusing on the articulation from the heel to the ball of the foot. The garden was not a large space, with a path that would take me maybe thirty seconds to walk around at a normal speed. But shadowing Toryo's pace, it took us an incredible fifteen minutes. That's how slow we were.

I had one hand on my heart, the other on my core, while Toryo explained how important it was to have awareness of your core and activate through the abs, which I loved, of course. Moving so slowly felt amazing and infuriating in equal measure; my lack of patience came in, and I had to say to myself, *Just relax. This is what you're here for, to take it in. What's the rush, Andrea?* It was then that I started to find more zen. I started to find more power in my breath, more awareness.

I knew I had to include awareness walking as a next-level option for Daily Practice #2, using concentrated steps as a form of mindful stretching.

## awareness walking

### WHAT IT DOES
Gently stretches the legs and torso and quiets the mind

### TIME IT TAKES
2 to 3 minutes or more

### HOW TO DO IT
Simply walk at a slow speed, allowing yourself to be hyperaware of every step, the roll of your foot from heel to toe, the subtle shifting of weight from leg to leg, while breathing calmly.

You may not be able to go for a long walk right when you wake up—though I recommend doing so if you can! Regardless of when you do it or how far you go, awareness walking brings many of the same benefits as your morning stretch and breathing exercises. For me, it is really a moving meditation. Let your mind relax as you walk. Don't call your friends; don't fret about dinner. Just let your mind wander as you take in your surroundings.

Albert Einstein, Virginia Woolf, and Ludwig von Beethoven all loved to walk, and they used that time to test and perfect their world-changing ideas. Even if you have humbler ambitions, a mindful walk can still have amazing benefits for your health and productivity. It doesn't have to be quite as slow as my walk with Toryo, but it can help you achieve a meditative state. I find stretching my legs via a walk an ideal pick-me-up when my energy is slumping, and it's how I dream up my best ideas. Head outside—no headphones—and get moving.

## Fancy Footwork

If you keep feeling yourself pulled back to thoughts of work or kids, pay attention to how your feet feel against the ground. Listen to the sound of your steps. This practice will help you learn to control your troubling thoughts, rather than letting them control you.

As I walked with Toryo, I realized how we're sometimes conscious of the pressure and weight in the front foot, but how often do we think about the shifting of balance between the front and back foot?

Bear with me on all this fancy foot stuff—I have a point here!

In that temple tea garden in Kyoto, walking in slow motion with Toryo, the modern monk, I realized that being aware of this natural movement was the perfect analogy for the motion of life.

We're either on our front foot or more on our back foot. Perhaps we're always aggressively moving forward or thinking how we can do better—how we can do more, earn more, have more. How can we keep pushing? Or, perhaps we're the opposite, mainly on our back foot and weighed down by the past, our disappointments, and our problems. Toryo showed me that to find that perfect gait and a way of walking with ease, you need an equal distribution of weight between the back and the front. By acknowledging that the back foot gives you stability, rooting you in the past; and the front foot is accelerating you along the path, pulling you toward the future—you will find that the sweet spot is right in between the two.

I will always cherish my time with Toryo and the lesson of how a situation I worried would feel too traditional and heavy was anything but. There was a lightness and sense of fun and discovery I hadn't anticipated, and I love how he helped strengthen my sense that stretching and movement have meditative effects

(I sometimes catch up with what he's doing online; it turns out he's also on Instagram).

Try each stretch routine, ideally after your morning breathwork, then decide which is your favorite and add it to your daily practice. Feel free to switch it up, focusing on different parts of your body: perhaps stretching dynamically during the weekdays and some extended awareness walking on weekends? And add in mantras about gratitude, purpose, and positivity if you like.

And that's Daily Practice #2: Stretch Yourself. Stretching for just three minutes toward health, happiness, and a long life—and secretly meditating while you do it, using a method delivered directly from Japan. You're welcome.

## daily practice #3

# just press play

*full-out effort and
mindful movement
to kick-start your day*

> **WHAT WILL I BE DOING?**
> A mindful mini workout with real intensity that's low impact, effective, and fun.
>
> **HOW LONG WILL IT TAKE?**
> Just 10 minutes, minimum.
>
> **WHEN DO I DO IT?**
> Each and every morning, right after breathwork and stretching.
>
> **AND WHAT WILL I ACHIEVE?**
> Increased energy, improved muscle tone, and a sense of well-being. You're going to feel like a superwoman! Through a series of simple exercises, you will discover your own personal challenge zone, create and sustain motivation, experience the proven antidepressant effect of contracting your muscles, and foster the longevity of a multimillion-dollar biohacker.

When I think about movement, I think about Pilates. And when I think about Pilates, I think about New York City. Joseph Pilates and his wife Clara opened their first studio in a tiny space on 8th Avenue just three blocks south of Central Park. It was 1926, the Roaring Twenties, and the United States was in the middle of a huge prosperity boom. The city became vibrant with art, fashion, theater, music, and money, and it was fizzing with creativity: it would have felt like the center of the universe. A century or so later, I get that same feeling whenever I return to New York. When I glimpse the city from the air, I have a visceral reaction; I can't quite put it into words, but when I finally arrive and walk the streets, block by block, it takes my breath away. I just feel alive.

Joseph and Clara's gym focused on what they called controlled movement, or Contrology, and under Clara's instruction (I love that Pilates has a long history of female instructors), the method became hugely popular with dancers and performers, like American stage icons Ruth St. Denis and Martha Graham, and even with writer Christopher Isherwood (whose novel *Goodbye to Berlin* inspired one of my favorite musicals, *Cabaret*). Contrology, which became Pilates, kickstarted a demand for specialized stretching and exercise. A *movement* movement, if you will.

I found I had a natural affinity for Pilates, and it soon became an essential part of my training and conditioning. It even made me feel a little closer to my own contemporary dance idols, Paula Abdul and Twyla Tharp (more on Tharp in a moment), who both practice Pilates. In the end, I just fell in love with it, and I became a Pilates instructor myself.

Through my Pilates studies and dance background, I know firsthand that motivation starts with physical activity. A short workout—even if you really don't feel like it—fires you up, ignites your interest and excitement, and makes it one thousand times more likely you'll do it all again tomorrow. Sure, we can work on our mindset, improve it with meditation and visualization, motivating ourselves to achieve our goals while sitting in stillness, but if you still feel mighty far away from enlightenment, nirvana, seventh heaven, or whatever we're calling it, there's another indispensable and transformative tool. It does demand a little grit. Just a tiny, tiny grain of it. Enough to get you up, into your workout clothes, and moving for ten minutes, which, incidentally, is the time it takes to scroll a handful of Stories on Instagram or brew and drink a cup of coffee.

So many women I work with have come to me because they want to start exercising but have, in the past, struggled with motivation. How could they get themselves over the line? I tell them what I'm telling you right now: just start small. And do it with consistency. Before they knew it, their motivation had returned, and they were bringing the same hope and determination to every other aspect of their lives.

And when I say small, I mean really small. Just ten minutes, in fact. And if you start there, setting yourself a mini goal, you can gather great momentum. Think of it as Newton's first law of habit formation: objects in motion tend to stay in motion. Ten minutes, when you're used to less, can only help you up your exercise game and lock in your other morning habits. So, once you have finished your breathwork and morning stretching, Daily Practice #3 is a quick and impactful workout—and it will have you feeling ready to take on the world (it really will!).

## How to Do It

So, what exactly are we doing? For Daily Practice #3, I want you to do a smart-thinking, smart-moving, very simple ten-minute exercise sequence that will challenge every part of your body: arms, legs, back, and core. Do something you know will make you feel hot and sweaty and say, "Wow, did I really just do that?" at the end. For now, avoid anything overcomplicated with a steep learning curve. Motivation will always come a little easier if you focus on what you love.

A ten-minute bodyweight circuit works perfectly here: a series of simple exercises from squats and lunges to planks and push-ups, with or without an exercise mat, and ten minutes gives you just enough time to repeat each circuit about three times. The sequence below is challenging, customizable, and so much fun, and ten minutes will be over before you know it.

A bodyweight circuit might look something like:

30 seconds of high knees at a fast pace
20 squats
10 push-ups, on your knees
20 jumping jacks
10 forward lunges, repeating for both legs
15 seconds of holding a plank, on your forearms and feet or knees

Repeat three times. Turn up the dial by slowing down during the harder parts and/or adding weights and speeding up the aerobic aspects (like those high knees and jumping jacks). Search online to find a low-impact routine you like the look of, and stick to it.

If you're a Pilates or Barre girl, do your best high-tempo routine (and don't skip those hundreds) until the timer hits ten minutes.

If your thing is running or cycling, then run or spin for ten minutes.

Love dance? Play your favorite dance workout video—yep, for ten minutes. That's three or four big pop anthems in a row, and there are a million free workouts on YouTube, Instagram, and TikTok, set to retro 1990s remixes, movie soundtracks, heavy metal to classical and show tunes—whatever gets you there.

And, if none of this is possible for you where you are right now, your Daily Practice #3 is a fast-paced walk. For just ten minutes. Again, think about ways you can make it more effective. So, if you love to walk, how can you make it more challenging? Could you carry arm weights in your hands? Can you walk on an incline? What can you do to amp it up and get something more out of it? The nonnegotiable here for your Daily Practice #3 is that it's a ten-minute session, minimum, and that it's challenging.

That *challenge* word is important. I want you to discover your own personal challenge zone. I want you to get your breath going and your muscles a little quivery and shaky. This is not meant to be a low-intensity workout, and nor should it be. It's low impact, sure, but in this session, you're going to kick your ass for ten minutes a day. That's it. You'll know you're putting in the right amount of effort when you're breathing heavy, feeling fatigued, maybe even sweating. I want you to think, *I can't believe that was only ten minutes—it feels like I just did an hour-long workout!*

Here's my framework for choosing your own Daily Practice #3 and keeping on track:

## The FEEL Framework

I have an easy four-letter acronym I share with all my clients. FEEL stands for Fast, Effective, Enjoyable, and Lifelong—and it is the key to sustainable and impactful exercise:

### *F Is for Fast*

You do not have to work out for more than ten minutes for big results. If you work out at high intensity—meaning you are pushing your endurance and strength to your fullest potential—you will improve your strength, stamina, flexibility, and coordination in less time than it takes to boil an egg.

### *E Is for Effective*

These workouts should activate every major muscle group, get results, and help you reach your potential in a brief amount of time. This kind of intense movement requires a deep coordination between your mind and your body and a focus on how you are moving. You need to be present in the moment if you are going to go full out on every rep. Some moves will feel challenging, even if they look basic on paper—but they work when you do the work.

## E Is for Enjoyable

This is so, so important: I want you to have fun. Many people see working out as a punishment or a chore, instead of one of the best things you can possibly do to improve your state of mind (and your physical health). If you dread your workouts, you'll likely look for ways to avoid them or cut them short—you won't be nearly as consistent. One of my friends loves online high-intensity workouts set to movie musical numbers like those in *The Greatest Showman*; you do you! Finding exercises that you enjoy is absolutely key for following through on your workout plans.

## L Is for Lifelong

Workouts should be challenging and even humbling at times, but they should never cause injury. You want them to be sustainable through all phases of your life, so prioritize exercises that focus on endurance, strength, and mobility. Be honest about where you are in your fitness journey. Even if you have to adapt your moves a bit, you can always keep coming back to them.

When I think about that last point, L is for Lifelong, I think about one of my clients, Judy. Nearly a decade ago, when I was living in Boca Raton, South Florida, Judy came to my class three times a week. She was older than most of her classmates, but just as focused, if not more so. Could she do everything the same as the twenty-one-year-old next to her? No. But you know what? She had better stamina than anyone. It was wild. And in our last session together, before I moved to New York City, she told me she was just shy of eighty and "in the best shape of my life." What I loved about her was her consistency. The effectiveness of her approach. And, of course, her positivity. If she couldn't do something, her attitude was: "So what? I'll modify." She showed up.

With every workout I do, I am pushing myself to my personal limit, where I know I will get the best physical and emotional results for my efforts. In what I call the "Challenge Zone," I not only overcome my fatigue for the last rep of my workout—I achieve an amazing moment of emotional release. If you push past whatever is holding you back and prove to yourself how capable you are of doing more than you thought possible, you will experience this catharsis, too. You will cultivate a new confidence and strength. Keep striving for your goals—because you can. (An important word of caution: Always be mindful when you are working out. If you are tired to the point where you can't keep your form, you are going too far—you will find an injury instead of catharsis!)

Working out, hard, for ten minutes every day, motivates you. It invites the attitude of "If I can do that, I can do anything." If you know you just nailed eight more reps of a plié than usual, and you were shaking and quivering as you did it, you can sure as heck take out the trash, finish that report, or write the next chapter of that book. When you prevail through those hard moments, you are reminded of what you are truly capable of.

Isn't that just what we teach our children? We give them experiences to discover failure, because it's through failure that they learn how to do the hard things and deal with them in the future. Without overcorrecting them, we give our kids these opportunities, because they need to learn—gently—where their own challenge zone is, and how they can push themselves a little further.

When I take my daughters to cheer practice (which is really a form of complex gymnastics) and look on from the bleachers, I see these kids repeat, repeat, repeat each amazing move right up until their form is wobbly. At that point, the coach knows it could become a safety issue, so they stop—but they've really challenged themselves up until that moment.

If you didn't get to do this as a kid, don't worry. Daily Practice #3 can be a game changer for any kind of emotional obstacle, including ones a lot more challenging than morning sleepiness. It gives you confidence in yourself—in your determination and self-regulation—when you can push all the negative thoughts to the side and follow through on the workout you know you need.

In other words, it's deeply therapeutic. In the most trying times I've been through, I've learned to just keep making small moves day in, day out. Soon, no matter what else is happening in my life, I'll start to feel a bit more in control.

## Not Wanting to Work Out . . . But Doing It Anyway

I need to underline my earlier point about motivation again because it's so important. Not wanting to do the thing—but doing it anyway—is key. When many people meet a "workout person," they think she wakes up every morning, just ready to go. *I wish!*

Okay, for me, it's partly true: sometimes I wake up totally excited for the day, but there are plenty—plenty—of other times I don't want to get out of bed at all. Even after years of daily workouts, I need a system I can fall back on when I simply want to go back to bed. For me, that's my morning breathwork and bedside stretching—it's a cue for the rest of my body to get ready for a burst of exercise. And after years of doing it, it's become a habit.

On those mornings when the bed is almost too cozy and comfortable to leave, I think about one of my idols, the great choreographer Twyla Tharp, and an early chapter of her culture-changing book, *The Creative Habit*. She sets the scene: early morning in New York City, a daily workout that simply must be done but it's at Pumping Iron gym, a cab ride away, and Twyla just does not feel like it. What's more, it's 5:30 AM.

"First steps are hard," she writes. "It's no one's idea of fun to wake up in the dark every day and haul one's tired body to the gym. Like everyone, I wake up, stare at the ceiling, and ask myself, Gee, do I feel like working out today?" For Twyla, it's the ritual of waving down a cab and telling the driver the destination that ensures her workout is going to happen. And that, for her, is the hardest part. Once she's at Pumping Iron, she knows she can complete her workout. It's committing to it—waving down the cab at 5:30 AM—that's the hard part. But the routine of actually getting out of bed, putting on her sweats, and heading out onto the street means she's going to achieve what she's set out to do. No doubt about it.

## Just Press Play

I know that not-wanting-to-do-this feeling so well, and so do many of the women I work with. When we're not really feeling our best, not really vibing it, unsure, or there's something holding us back, to those women, and to myself, I always say: Just Press Play.

When I am about to start my exercise routine, I visualize pushing the triangular play button on my phone screen. If you are nostalgic, you can picture the play button on your old iPod, your long-lost Discman, even your boom box of yore—whatever gives you a jump.

Just Press Play has become a catchphrase for my fitness and coaching clients and my followers (I even trademarked it!), but the point is to have a simple and inspiring mantra you can say when you need it.

As a dancer in training, I had to be ready to start moving whenever I heard the instructor count us in with the words "five, six, seven, eight." A four count does not leave much time for self-doubt! When my dance teacher started counting, I knew I had to be ready to go. If you find yourself overthinking—and you want a variation on Just Press Play—try counting off five, six, seven, eight, and go!

So many of my happiest, most successful clients start right here, on just ten minutes a day. Many upgrade, eventually feeling confident to go further, and join my thirty-minute workouts over at BODi.com and go on to do more and more.

But, at the beginning, all that's important to me is that they start; they Just Press Play with a simple, ten-minute workout, every single day. I don't care if that's where you're at for six months or more, or if ten minutes is your long-term sweet spot. I just want you to start.

I want you to start because I know those minutes add up. At the end of week one, you'll have worked out at a high intensity for a total of seventy minutes. And the more consistently you do it—oh my gosh—the changes are tremendous! You will start to feel better. You will have more energy. You're going to see muscle tone. You're going to be stronger. You're going to have energy that you never had before. Your endorphins are going to be spiking. And suddenly, you're going to feel like a superwoman.

## Hope Is in the Muscles

Working out has incredible physical benefits on top of the emotional ones, of course. Do Daily Practice #3 just once, and you'll achieve a rush of happy endorphins. Do it frequently, and you'll discover renewed strength and you'll have a healthier cardiovascular system—even for only a quick burst of daily activity. If you don't think you do already, you'll look amazing, and you'll feel amazing, too.

The physical benefits of movement—especially short bursts of challenging exercise—are endless. It can help us heal from major injury, or even improve some chronic illnesses like respiratory and cardiovascular diseases, lowering the risk of diabetes, stroke, and perhaps even dementia. Working out at a high intensity for ten minutes has roughly the same fitness effect as an hour-long steady walk. Challenging your muscles with something like strength training burns fat long after you've ended your session, even as it builds muscle, and more muscle means you can consume more calories. What's more, exercise increases blood flow to the surface of the skin (if you have lighter skin, you'll have noticed a pink-red flush), oxygenating and nourishing, bringing healing and improving skin quality over time.

We all know that moving makes us feel good. But, in 2021, researchers at the Medical University of Vienna found literal evidence. Like, it really, truly makes you feel good! Meet the focus of their study, myokines, aka "hope molecules." They're the mysterious chemicals, proteins, or peptides (depending on what study you read) that are released into the bloodstream when our muscles contract. Some myokines cross the blood-brain barrier, and there, they do something amazing: they give us a little but measurable mood lift. Incredibly, these myokines act as antidepressants, improving our mood, knowledge absorption, and even helping stave off inflammation and brain aging. The researchers' study focused on ways to combat "late-life depression," pointing out that although we already know exercise is good for our mental health, "the underlying mechanisms are still poorly understood." Their findings were fascinating; the researchers think there really could be something in these hope molecules (which is such an unscientific-sounding term, but I'm totally here for it), which were found to be more common in athletes than in a test group.

Shortly after that study was published, a team of number crunchers at the University of Potsdam took the idea that exercise might combat depression—and supersized it. They undertook a huge systematic review of forty-one different studies across thousands of human subjects, and in 2023 in the *British Medical Journal*, they revealed that, yes, exercise can be used as medicine for depressive symptoms.

"We found large, significant results," said lead exercise scientist Andreas Heissel, to *The Washington Post* in 2023, taking pains to make it clear you don't have to go crazy to achieve positive effects. No one's asking you to sign up for an ultramarathon or do a set of one-arm pull-ups (unless you're reading this book with your other hand, of course). But something—ten minutes of movement a day—is better than nothing. In fact, Heissel's team's work was so compelling that the National Health Service in the United Kingdom changed its guidance for treating mild and moderate depression from prescribing antidepressants to—you guessed it—exercise!

That idea, that exercise is medicine, thrills me. What it tells me is that there's hope, not just in those molecules, but locked inside our own muscles. And I love the idea that every single squat or lunge, every bicep curl or ab crunch, every unscrewing of the peanut butter jar, might truly spark a tiny but not insignificant happy feeling. And who doesn't want that?

Now, imagine doing all this with consistency. Each and every day. Girl, for the time it takes to scroll a few Stories on Instagram, you could do ten sweaty minutes of happy-making movement!

## Ready for More? Let's Upgrade Your Workout!

As I mentioned earlier, Daily Practice #3 can be a health-saver, but it's also a starting point: so many of my clients go on to do longer and more challenging workouts. That's because those small moves add up and, before long, you will probably find those ten minutes are just the minimum your body needs. As you get fitter, stronger, and more motivated, you might want to go further, progressing into more complex sessions. This is certainly true of Sarah, one of my Xtend Barre clients. We'll get to her story in a moment, but she used small moves—moves she thought seemed nearly impossible to achieve at one time—to upgrade her workout and truly transform her life.

If you work from home, spend most of your days at the computer, and desperately need social interaction (like me!), then make it a mission to seek out a local studio. It could be a regular gym, a local Pilates studio, or a small fitness center. If you're new to working out outside of the home, then I highly recommend finding a smaller boutique-type of studio that will offer a more intimate vibe. Once you find your workout place, it often begins to feel like a second home, and you can't wait to catch up with new friends (accountability partners!) and look forward to this time in your day to focus just on you.

Or maybe you are more of an introvert and enjoy working out solo? Seek out some great at-home online workouts or a coach you admire on social media to see if they can do private one-on-one sessions via Zoom. For now, just focus on those ten minutes, every day; that's what's important here.

## Modifying Your Moves

As I might have mentioned, I love a retreat, and as I write this book, I am putting together the finishing touches on my next one. I'm especially excited to finally meet one of my online Pilates clients, Claudia, in person for the first time. In her mid-thirties, she suffered a major seizure that almost killed her. When she woke up in the hospital, it became clear that some movement in her arm and wrist was permanently disabled, and her shoulder was affected, too. Claudia knew she could improve things through mobility exercises, and she used Xtend Barre to do it. I designed XB as a full-body workout and, well, it's not easy; it really puts you in your challenge zone. But Claudia consistently shows up, rethinking and then modifying any move her body can't quite do (yet).

What I love about this is that she never lets these modifications define her or thinks, *This exercise just isn't for me.* She never sits out a single move. I knew none of her background when we first spoke after class, although I'd noticed how cleverly she transitioned between positions, and how hard she pushed herself. "You just flow through, modify, and never stop!" I said. It was then that she told me about her journey, how she had modified many of the XB moves to suit her mobility, and we spoke about what she was hoping to achieve long-term. I was so in awe. Many of us in that position would have said, "Nope, not for me; I can't do that kind of workout anymore," but not Claudia.

It got me thinking about how easily we can sit things out, how we can let the inertia-loving part of our brains help us find the right excuse, from "I've got a sniffle" to "I'm too tired." But Claudia's inner voice had said, "Absolutely not—I'm going to figure a way around this and make sure I can still participate." We all have different limitations, but Claudia has taught herself to approach hers creatively. Thinking on your feet like this takes a huge amount of energy, and I often think of Claudia as one of the hardest-working XB women I know.

## Give Yourself a Lift

As you build strength and stamina through your short, intense daily workouts, there's something I want you to have on your radar, something that will ultimately make you more resilient, powerful, and age-proof: I want you to prioritize resistance training. I'm talking barbells, free weights or machines in the gym, resistance bands, and even bodyweight exercises (where you work against the weight of your own body—like in the sample circuit on page 65). Yes, lifting weights hasn't always been thought of as a women's workout, but if we continue to think of weight training as a male domain, we will be missing out on something essential for our long-term health.

Our muscle mass grows steadily from birth throughout our teens and twenties, and peaks for most of us around the age of thirty-five. From that point, with no intervention, our strength gradually diminishes at a slow, comfortable rate until approximately sixty-five years old (for women, and seventy for men) when the process generally speeds up. At this point, any physical power we've lost along the way starts to make itself known through increased risk of injury, obesity, bone-density loss, and even falling. It doesn't have to be this way. If we build up a base of muscle through strength training, we'll not only be stronger and fitter, but we'll also be insuring ourselves against age-related problems in the future.

You don't have to lift super heavy weights (unless that's your thing!). Lifting light weights with higher repetitions has a similar effect to lifting heavy weights with fewer reps, in that both increase muscle mass. But there is a difference: light weights/high reps helps to enhance muscle endurance, while heavy weights/fewer reps improves overall strength.

But what I really love about resistance training is that the more we demand of our muscles, the faster we burn through our reserves of adenosine triphosphate (ATP), a miracle molecule responsible for delivering energy to our cells. And the more we burn through our ATP, the more our bodies replenish it, meaning positive outcomes not only for our muscles but for every cell in our bodies. Our metabolism gets a boost, we'll burn calories more efficiently (for hours, even days, after our resistance workouts), abdominal fat can also decrease, previously high blood pressure can lower, and some research even suggests our bone density might increase. So, if you're not already doing so, start to add weights or body-weight exercises to your daily workouts and give yourself a lift.

## Beating the Biohack Bros

In the past few years, from the sidelines, I've watched the biohack industry grow from a few fringe studies to a full-blown wellness movement. Today, biohacking—supercharging your health through small lifestyle moves: dietary, fitness, and even medical and technical tweaks—is big business. According to *Fortune*, it amounts to $26 billion, in fact, and it's set to grow even bigger. It has its own elite products and costly supplements, exclusive programs and retreats, bespoke gene analyses, and even its own multimillion-dollar superstars, almost all men—the biohack bros.

As a genre of health research, it's fascinating, I admit. Some of these industry figures who are spending millions of dollars testing their ideas on themselves and documenting their discoveries are real pioneers. And if biohacking means we can live longer, better, and happier, I'm all for it. But, considering the $255 vitamin subscriptions, expensive body scans, and endless Insta-ads, I also realized I had grown tired of all the posturing.

When Julie Gibson Clark stepped into the ring, it was like a breath of fresh air. In 2024, the fifty-five-year-old working single mom in Phoenix was revealed to be the world's number two in something called the Rejuvenation Olympics. It's an online international leaderboard of around four thousand people, many of them biohackers, who medically track the pace at which they biologically age. Without the supplements, scans, and gadgets, without the multimillion-dollar budget, and without the time to biohack herself, even Julie was surprised.

But, as *Fortune* reported, other women like Julie had a few things in common. First, biohacking and the biohacker bros don't impress them much. Me either. Instead, they were "defining longevity goals in their own terms," and many said they were motivated by a "desire to stick around for those [they] love and care for."

Considering herself "health conscious" in general, with daily sessions of movement and meditation, and eating lots of vegetables, Julie shared her solid-gold insights in an interview with journalist Alexa Mikhail. One line really stood out to me. On hearing her position on the leaderboard, and after her initial shock, Julie said it "confirmed this stuff has to just kind of be like brushing your teeth."

This idea *really* resonates with me, as it's something I know to be true myself. I know from experience that doing something small, each and every day, can have huge benefits.

I always say: small moves, big life.

Small, daily practices done as consistently as brushing your teeth can give you the health of a multimillionaire biohacker.

## Starting Where You Are

Dancing can be the highest of highs. Just before the music starts, you're in position, buzzing with anticipation; you're controlling your breath and feeling all those lovely, healthy nerves—it's intoxicating. It's how I imagine a comedian feels when the whole stadium laughs, or a singer when they hit that hard-to-reach note: that's just how it is when a dancer takes to the stage. When I stopped dancing professionally, I knew I had to find that high again. How could I keep movement in my life?

It's rare for physical performers to dance their way into their thirties, forties, and beyond, and like a professional athlete whose career is usually over when they're still young, it's hard not to get the retirement blues! Thank goodness I was able to segue my love for movement into Pilates and fitness.

When I started to teach and help others reach their fitness goals, a little bit of that high came back. Being in front of a class, watching people move their bodies, helping them move and find their motivation—it felt good! Leaving the dance world, I thought I'd left real live performance behind, but years later, as a super trainer, I ended up performing in front of the biggest live audience of my life.

It took a decade of small moves to find my way onto BODi, a leading online fitness platform, but I made it and was soon invited to the company's annual summit. That meant three days of talks, group workouts, appearances, and all things fitness at a huge venue in St. Louis. The first thing I noticed were the crowds: some ticket holders were lining up by 4 AM to get the best spot for the main-stage class and to finally meet the trainers they had been training with online for months. Every person there had movement on their mind.

I'd already built Xtend Barre and had worked hard on raising my profile, but, apart from studio classes, intimate events, and retreats, I didn't yet know if anyone had really heard of Andrea Leigh Rogers. That all changed when I was introduced as a super trainer on stage. There, I taught a class of twelve hundred, and at the main-stage event, there were more than thirteen thousand people in the audience, all cheering and mirroring my every move. It was the highest of highs. Although the nerves were there (I love those healthy, full-of-anticipation, I'm-doing-something-big nerves), once I take stage, something happens—they fade away and I know I am right where I am supposed to be. I call that feeling "the extraordinary ordinary!"

Imagine it: Thousands of people working out together, all moving together. There's this high energy in the room; it's full of endorphins, and afterward everyone wants your picture—you feel like a rock star! It more than filled the absence I'd felt since the end of my dancing career.

We all start from a different place. You might have lapsed from a usual regular workout routine, and your health—mental and physical—might already be great and you just want to improve. For others, this is all pretty new—the last time they truly worked out was in their high school gym class. And for a few, they might be in a very low place in their life—somewhere most of us have visited at one point or another—where even just reading this chapter is a challenge. I get it.

## Kickstarting Your Motivation

One of the best things about my career is connecting with women all over the world, just like Sarah, a nurse practitioner in her mid-thirties, with whom I first spoke in August 2022. She reached out to me on Instagram with a simple, friendly message. "Hey, Andrea," she typed, "I'm doing your Xtend Barre program and I'm loving it, here's where I'm at . . ." and we just started connecting. She was going through some challenges at the time, and I loved talking to her. Two years later I am just in awe of Sarah's commitment and dedication to her health, both physical and mental, and the emotional journey that she's been on. Also, she's smart. Like, really smart.

An aspect of my work is designing and curating a series of fitness and health programs for my brand, Xtend Barre, just like the one Sarah did. Although most women do the program from home, there's lots of accountability, a Facebook group, live sessions, and every week or so we hold regular XB group check-ins online where the community shares news, advice, support, and encouragement. Around the time I was writing this book, I invited Sarah along to tell her story.

There are quite a few of us in the community, and that morning, a number of fantastic women dialed in. Seeing into other women's lives and hearing where they're at—mentally and physically—is always a pleasure, and I know the other women think so, too: so many are regulars. Some quietly take notes; others ask clever questions. One woman cleans her entire home from top to bottom with her AirPods in. Another does what looks like an endless stream of laundry (which is folded perfectly by the end of the session), and another is often at her desk in a busy office, doing her work, but with our discussion going on in the background; all of us are busy women who can clearly do more than one thing at a time.

I asked Sarah to share her story of how she transformed her health and lost over one hundred pounds in two years. I remember she was glowing, radiating this extreme joy at discovering herself again. Even her posture was on point (we love to talk about posture in my classes and in these sessions; it's my thing), something that deserved some praise, right off.

Sarah laughed. "That's probably, you know, what XB programs have really helped me with: my grounding, my posture, my balance, flexibility and mobility, just feeling stable and strong. I'm so thankful for that because now I can just be proud and upright and share it with everybody." I remember her charming everyone on that call as she told her story.

A few years earlier, Sarah had had emergency eye surgery and, while it was successful, the aftercare was tough. "You have to be bed bound or couch bound," she explained. "You cannot be up and moving because of the healing process." But what was supposed to be a three-month or less healing period turned into about nine months. "I was unable to move my body more than five minutes every hour. And I struggled. My health and my mental health were just broken, very, very broken. [I was at] 265 pounds. I couldn't walk up the stairs. My joints were killing me, and I could barely breathe."

Things improved when she was allowed to move again, but then other medical challenges presented themselves. She was diagnosed with polycystic ovary syndrome (PCOS), prediabetes, and high cholesterol, and when she was told she needed to lose weight if she wanted to safely have children, she was devastated. "So, after having my eye [problem], and then having all these health diagnoses, it was like, 'I can't do this [commit to a healthy lifestyle]. This is too hard,'" said Sarah. "I almost accepted that this is what my life was going to be."

So many of us can relate to that feeling. When everything seems to be just piling on, bad thing after bad thing, catastrophe after catastrophe. Eventually, a tiny voice inside you says, *Why try?* It's a you-can't-do-this-you're-not-worthy-you-don't-have-what-it-takes kind of voice. And you think, *Why try? It's too hard. I'm not going to get out of this.*

When Sarah and I were first in touch, knowing nothing of her situation, we sent Sarah a surprise invite to join the full Xtend Barre test program, and it flipped a switch. "Getting that invitation was like, 'Okay, I got to do this. I can't give up. I have to do this,'" said Sarah. "I think another switch . . . was that I'm a health care provider, and I have to tell people what they need to do for their health. How can I tell somebody to do that when I'm not doing that myself?"

And underneath all of this was something else driving Sarah, something too powerful to ignore: "I really wanted to have kids, and I didn't want to die. That's it." We were all a little quiet in that moment, allowing Sarah's words to sink in.

"Were you in the mindset to do it?" I asked Sarah.

"No," she laughed. "Did I want to quit and give up right when I got that invite? Absolutely. But I thought, 'You know what, you're going to be working so closely with everybody; you need this accountability.' I knew that if I didn't get up and do [each session], I was going to get a DM: 'Sarah, where are you? Why did you do this?'" And so, she thought, *Stop, no more excuses. This is for your health.* Soon, the positive voice overruled the negative one.

With so much warmth, honesty, and humor, Sarah told us how she did it. Just like Julie Gibson Clark winning out over the biohack bros, she got there with small daily actions, consistency, and a positive mindset. She wondered, "How am I going to make it through a workout?" But she did. "I didn't pass out and I didn't die! I was like, 'Oh my God, I can do this!'" So, she did it again.

Her determination, day in, day out, eventually saw her lose five pounds. She told herself, "Great. Let's get to seven pounds," and then, "Great. Let's get to ten pounds." And when she got to ten, she said, "Maybe I can do this. And then I got to fifteen, and fifteen turned into twenty, and then it just kept going, and that was really when I started feeling that grit and determination in myself. And I was like, 'No, twenty is not good enough. I want to be able to run!' I just kept mini goal setting. And when I hit that goal, I was like, 'Wow! Okay, next goal!'"

I think I screamed a little when Sarah mentioned "mini goals." I definitely got goose bumps. Doing small actions, each and every day—that's exactly what I'm preaching. In these online XB sessions, my classes, my coaching sessions and talks, even to my family and friends, I'm always saying the same thing: small moves, big life. And I say small moves, big life, because it takes those dedicated small steps to make a big change.

If a doctor said you had to lose a hundred pounds, it would seem impossible. A mountain trail so steep and far reaching, it seems unthinkable to climb on your own. But Sarah did it. And she did it through mini goals, step by step, through small moves to build a big life.

There's something else going on here, too. Something I think of as the cycle of motivation. Sarah explained that achieving these mini goals made her feel good and—in conjunction with small but obvious improvements in her health—her "mental game kind of switched up a little bit." Every single day you Just Press Play on your challenge, your workout, your job, or any small, boring chore is a moment of you doing a hard thing you really didn't want to do. And yet, you did it, so you feel accomplished; you feel pride. Doing the thing is a motivator.

## Movement Snacks

My favorite ways to supplement a daily exercise routine are with short jolts of body-friendly activity I call "movement snacks." This is not in lieu of a ten-minute intensive workout and does not need to be done in sequence in the morning—let it simply liven up your day whenever an opportunity presents itself.

So, what the heck is a movement snack? Kinesiology researchers at Canada's McMaster University call short bursts of exercise interspersed throughout the day "exercise snacks." For me, "exercise" may even be taking it too far! It is just about moving your body when you have a quiet moment (or when the feeling moves you). They're not wind sprints—a movement snack can be a pre-Zoom yoga pose, a post-lunch stretch, or heel lifts while I am folding the laundry. The researchers showed that these "snacks" have the same benefits as more strenuous exercise, including strengthening your cardiovascular system and muscles.

Here are just some of the many small exercises I do almost every day:

Pliés (knee bends) as I brush my teeth
Push-ups at the bathroom and/or kitchen counter as I wait
    for the microwave to ding.

Walking squats around the house while on a phone call
Lunges, squats, and heel lifts while cooking
Stretches between Zoom meetings
A short trampoline jumping series during TV commercials (yes, I have a mini tramp in my living room)
Heel lifts while folding laundry
Torso side twists while seated at my desk
Planks with my kids (we see who can hold it the longest!)
Currently doing squats as I review and edit this book!

Sarah pointed out that it wasn't until she started to see and feel results that her mind and motivation caught up with her. Did Sarah want to do those first few workout sessions? No, but she did them anyway. The action of doing them made things better, which, in turn, motivated her to do more. Don't wait for motivation to come; just tell yourself, *Okay, girl, get your ass up and let's do this, right? Let's actually do this!*

The group had so many questions, and one woman asked Sarah how she keeps on track—surely, she must have had times when she wanted to quit?

She thought about it for a moment and then said:

"You can fall off the wagon; just don't set up camp."

I just love that analogy! In the moment, I could see the rest of the group taking it in, too. Slowly, smiles spread across everyone's faces. After that zinger, Sarah went on: "Maybe you haven't worked out for a week? Just acknowledge it, feel the feels, and move the heck on."

It's okay to fail, to fall off the wagon, but we're not building a campfire and singing "Kumbaya"; we're getting back on and continuing our journey—due north, right? I remember feeling wowed! "Oh, I'm using that one, Sarah," I said. "I think that is a beautiful way of really visualizing those little setbacks."

Just like Sarah receiving her invite to class, *when* in your life you pick up this book is important. For her, it was the right time to start her journey, and she soon found that movement motivated her. Onscreen at our XB meet-up, Sarah sparkled: she came across like the success story she truly is. Sometimes, when we see someone do so well, it's okay to admit to a little uneasiness. It's hard not to compare ourselves with women like Sarah who have achieved so much. But, as she pointed out in our session, she didn't get there overnight, but by meeting mini goal after mini goal, ten minutes by ten minutes, until she had two years and one hundred pounds behind her.

We must remember that we all emerge at different times. So it might not be your time today, but finding your challenge zone and moving for just ten minutes—each and every day—will ensure you get there. Stick to the trail because your time to shine is coming; I just know it.

Until then, got ten minutes to spare?

Let's get sweaty, get our heart rate up, and feel the burn.

―――― **daily practice #4** ――――

# do the thing

*a radical approach
to daily productivity*

> **WHAT WILL I BE DOING?**
> Completely rethinking your to-do list.
>
> **HOW LONG WILL IT TAKE?**
> Just 2 minutes.
>
> **WHEN DO I DO IT?**
> After your morning moves.
>
> **AND WHAT WILL I ACHIEVE?**
> You will scale down your to-do list, identify your nonnegotiables, and actually achieve what you really need to do. "But there's too much on my to-do list already!" I hear you—and that's why we're changing things up and completely refocusing. It's a heady feeling, believe me. It all starts with ripping up what's gone before and giving yourself a break. Are you ready? Let's Do The Thing.

Let's hear it for the frazzled. Those multitasking, multiskilled superhero women (come on, they're almost always women) whose days are filled with countless tasks and to-dos. Balancing work and family or caring responsibilities, studying in between taxiing their loved ones to swim meets, vet appointments, and birthday parties; they are somehow everything to everyone and are doing well even if they are just keeping it all together. Even then, these high achievers are often haunted by "mom guilt" (more on that later in this chapter), their own untapped potential, and those last-minute World Book Day kids' costumes they have to make tonight before fixing tomorrow's school lunches. Procrastination? They don't even have time for it.

Daily Practice #4 is a radical approach to simplifying your life and starting to conquer those frazzled feelings. Much like "Just Press Play," "Do The Thing" (or #DTT) is a no-nonsense way to cut through all the overthinking and do what really needs to be done. When it comes to productivity, I consider it my blueprint for success. I've practiced it for years and could not have achieved half of what I have without it. Now, I'll admit, it's a little counterintuitive, but hear me out!

Do The Thing is shorthand for my favorite riff on the to-do list, that daunting catch-all for everything you have been putting off doing. I know a to-do list can help, but if you are like me, it is far from a perfect solution.

Sometimes, when life is too chaotic or I am finding myself overstressed, the to-do list becomes a barrier between me and decisive, productive activity. Writing out a list of tasks is supposed to calm and order the mind, but sometimes there's just too much to do and I'm left feeling overwhelmed and anxious. In those moments, I can't *even*.

Noting down everything I have to achieve—including all the intimidating nitty-gritty of taking care of the house and my business, organizing work trips and my girls' schedules—means I just want to call it a day before the day has begun. What's even worse: I feel guilty about it. And if I'm not careful, this guilt eats away at my motivation, and I'm stuck in a forever cycle of not quite achieving.

So many of the women I work with have the same experience. With all the multitasking they do—for their families, home, and work—they're frazzled. Given a spare minute, they end up procrastinating what matters most to them. They're doing everything, yet nothing meaningful feels like it ever gets done, and in the meantime the list keeps growing.

In 2019, I was moving my family to New York City, going through a tough separation, organizing schooling and childcare, and restructuring my still-fragile business—I was trying to do it all. I had been in the process of rebuilding my life post-divorce for some time, and the New York move—a final but integral part of my plan—had been meticulously thought out. As we set off, I remember feeling that I was between two worlds. Of course, flying always underlines that strange, exciting sensation: after all, you are literally on your way from one place to another and you know things are about to change, whether in a small or significant way. But this time I was truly leaving one world behind, knowing another was about to be discovered.

I remember seeing New York from the air—a city I have always loved—and feeling intense anticipation and exhilaration. It was a feeling I recognized from that moment just before countless dance performances and auditions, the first time I took the stage for Disney, or when I led live exercise classes for thousands of attendees at the BODi expo. That fizzing feeling meant life was about to change—and for the better.

I knew I was doing the right thing, and I also knew, after some challenging years, I could truly rely on myself. But here I was managing the entire household on my own, playing both mom and dad to my girls. We had just moved across the country, and there were countless boxes to unpack (how were all these boxes going to fit into our tiny apartment?), and what the heck were we going to have for dinner? In short, I soon became completely overwhelmed!

Even as I checked items off my to-do list, it never seemed to get shorter, and I was having trouble simply tracking both my short- and long-term goals, much less reaching them. I wondered how I could be so busy and yet not really be getting anything done.

In the end, I had to admit my to-do list just wasn't working. Tasks that were initially important soon became urgent and then absolutely essential, and they just weren't getting crossed off. And this was not making me feel good, not at all. It undermined my sense of self. I had always thought of myself as a doer: even from a young age, skipping dance practice was unthinkable, and as a single mom and business owner, my world was powered by pulling myself together and getting shit done. In New York City, I could see the brightest future for my girls and me, but I just couldn't come up for air—and it felt like everything was on the line. I knew I needed a reset, a new strategy that would help me set clearer intentions, so success would look like . . . success, instead of merely not drowning.

I remember thinking, *Girl, you have to start to articulate what really needs to get done today because there's just too much and, if you're not careful, you're going to sink.*

And so this is how Do The Thing—sometimes known as Get Shit Done depending on my mood and how much I have to do—came out of my endless roster of tasks, aka the chaotic spectacle of Andrea Leigh Rogers and the Never-Ending To-Do List.

With what felt like hundreds (thousands?) of things I needed to achieve, I decided to do something truly radical.

I ripped up my to-do list.

And whoa, did it feel good!

## Getting Shit Done

After tossing my to-do list in the trash, I then took out a fresh sheet of paper. Only this time, I allowed myself to write down just three things: my most urgent items, the ones that would bring me the most satisfaction if I could only get them done. At the time, they were likely something like: finalize the new franchise agreement, review legal documents, and update passport. Numbered #1, #2, and #3, these were my nonnegotiables.

While anything on your "to-do list" is "to be done" sooner rather than later, these were actions I had to take that day, no excuses. I told myself, no matter what, come hell or high water, I was going to do these three things. And then, after I'd done each thing, I decided not to just quickly cross it off and move on, I wanted to really feel it. I took a moment to mindfully enjoy my achievement, and—because I love to self-motivate and I don't care who hears it—I said to myself, "Atta girl!"

I drew a box around my three nonnegotiables, and underneath I wrote down two "bonus round" tasks that would be a relief to check off. If I could get to tasks four and five, great! But I promised I wouldn't beat myself up if I ran out of time. One of my aims was to escape that looming feeling of always letting myself down and, with the natural mood lift that comes from achieving my goals, I knew that after doing my nonnegotiables, it would be likely I'd feel like doing more.

*Can I complete two more tasks?* I wondered.

Sure, I could.

And then, as I was really winning that day, I added one more task on the next line down. This would be one more activity, but something fun I could do for myself. It could be taking a nap on a summer afternoon, lighting a special candle for an evening bath, or trying a new face mask.

I saw that I'd created a reverse pyramid with my three nonnegotiables at the top, my two other to-dos on the next line down as bonuses, and then a final, single fun assignment at the bottom. The point of the final item is that it is something to look forward to and to make your whole list feel easier to approach. *Achieve your three nonnegotiables and you're a rock star*, I thought. *Achieve your nonnegotiables and your other tasks? Girl, you're not just a rock star, you're headlining.*

And so, that's just what I did.

From day one, I was amazed by how much lighter I felt.

Reading my to-do list no longer involved a tiring series of micro-decisions (can I put off doing X? what happens if I do Y before Z?). I had my marching orders, and I got to work. Day by day, my productivity ticked up, and I was able to take on ever more ambitious tasks while making definite progress toward my goals.

Here's the counterintuitive bit: doing less helped me do more.

Soon, my short-term daily list led me to a long-term mindset, and by simplifying my list to the most essential items, I could strategize about how I was using my time, forgive myself for the many things I would not have time to do (this was a real game changer: no more anxiety, guilt, and self-doubt), and celebrate that I was achieving what I set out to do, day after day.

Pleasingly, science backs me up. According to the *MIT Sloan Management Review*, "The power of specific, ambitious goals to improve the performance of individuals and teams is one of the best documented findings in organizational psychology and has been replicated in more than 500 studies over the past 50 years." This is just what I'd found by ripping up my to-do list and replacing it with fewer but more specific tasks!

One of the biggest benefits of simplifying your list this way—if you are no longer multitasking, jumping around, or skipping ahead—is that you can give each task full-out effort. Full-out effort was something I learned very early on in life. If my dance teacher said, "Mark it," she wanted us to walk through each move of a new dance in sequence. When she said, "Full out," she was telling us to give it absolutely everything we had, perform it with the most effort we could give. We knew we had to bring it. I feel the same way now when I need to get down to business—it has become my personal philosophy. I see it as part of a crucial equation, one that I'd love you to memorize: Consistency plus full-out effort plus time (because we often forget it takes time to get there) equals results.

### Consistency + Full-Out Effort + Time = Results

If you show up every day and you give it your all on just your three nonnegotiables, you will achieve results you never could have dreamed up. The key to both—for me—is my #DTT list.

## Procrastination and Its Drag-You-Down Effects

For a select few, putting things off and doing them at the very last possible moment with no time to spare is part of their creative process and, oddly, it's sometimes a successful strategy. There are award-winning novelists who identify as pantsers, meaning their approach to novel-writing is to fly by the seat of their pants rather than methodically plan and plot their work. Leonardo da Vinci took sixteen years to finish the *Mona Lisa*, and even

Mozart was known for his love of partying followed by eleventh-hour all-nighters (case in point: he delivered the overture to *Don Giovanni* with moments to spare, ink still wet—even after a fourteen-day extension!). While we're not all creative geniuses, running a house, business, and/or family can sometimes feel like an impossible feat, so it's comforting to know that even the greats struggled with procrastination, too.

It's something we're all familiar with, but there are those for whom procrastination is actively harmful. Not clearing your to-do list might leave you in a constant cycle of unease, which can lead to anxiety and, ultimately, the physical effects of stress. We're talking poor mental health, depression, and anxiety—even chronic conditions, specifically (and surprisingly) arm pain, according to a study published in 2023 by Fred Johansson, Alexander Rozental, and Klara Edlund of Sophiahemmet University in Stockholm. They analyzed data from thousands of subjects, all university students, to see if procrastination has associated health problems. News flash: it sure does.

Out of 3,525 Swedish university students, procrastination meant worse mental health and was associated with "unhealthy lifestyle behaviours (poor sleep quality and physical inactivity), and worse levels of psychosocial health factors (higher loneliness and more economic difficulties)" and a mysterious "disabling pain in the upper extremities." As other scientists weighed in on the research, they wondered if these physical and mental health problems were the cause of students putting things off, or the result.

What this tells me is that we must look at procrastination as part of a cycle. The more we don't Do The Thing, the more our health suffers, we lose motivation, and the less likely we are to achieve our goals; it's self-perpetuating. Much like "Just Press Play" and the idea that working out, even when we don't really feel like it, kickstarts our motivation, procrastination has the opposite effect.

Recently, a man I'll call Theo reached out to me during one of my online group coaching sessions. "I just procrastinate," he said, "and I always put things off, especially when I have to make phone calls, like the doctor or my insurance company or whatever it is, I just put it off."

I told Theo—and the rest of the attendees—to just think and do. When the idea to Do The Thing appears in your mind, acknowledge it (give it a quick nod), then just do it, there and then. Think and do, no questions asked. There's an issue of scale here, because if you're in quite a good place, you'll have the energy to do more, and your three big DTT things could be really, really big things. But sometimes you're overwhelmed, and just making that one annoying phone call is a huge accomplishment. When Theo told us that making these calls was his Achilles' heel, it set the chat room on fire! Almost all the other attendees said they hated making phone calls, too, but they also talked about how good it feels when you achieve something as seemingly insignificant as making a doctor's appointment. Focusing on that feeling and seeking to make it part of your everyday means you are no longer going to be that person who procrastinates.

That said, getting shit done isn't at all simple for much of the population. Many of us struggle with executive functioning as part of a disability, chronic illness, or neurodivergence. When it comes to attention and decision-making issues, even a late-in-life diagnosis can be transformative in helping to navigate the world. If you think you might benefit from a more formal assessment and a little more time and space to understand your needs, please put this book down right now and make an appointment for that evaluation.

I suggested to the group, and we decided together, collectively, that we were no longer going to be in that mindset. No longer were we going to define ourselves as people who don't make phone calls. We're the people who get shit done. (FYI: Theo messaged me later saying he'd finally made the call and felt a huge sense of relief—way to go, Theo!)

## How to Do It

To get started, open a clean notebook. I like to write in pen on real paper, because it is way too easy to edit or erase what you write on your phone or laptop, and there is just something especially satisfying about checking off an item on a handwritten list (I prefer to use a beautiful little notebook and pen; it just makes me feel happy). In fact, we might remember things more effectively when we write by hand.

## DO THE THING

In 2024, Ruud van der Weel and Audrey van der Meer, of the Developmental Neuroscience Lab at Norwegian University of Science and Technology, published a small study that seemed to show that writing by hand is uniquely powerful. Their high-density EEG study had students wear 256 electrodes to measure their brain activity when both handwriting on paper and typewriting on a screen and found that handwriting leads to "widespread brain connectivity."

The professors were interested in how traditional handwriting is being replaced by smartphone note apps, screenwork, and texting, and found, "When writing by hand, brain connectivity patterns were far more elaborate than when typewriting on a keyboard." Because of recent research, we know these "elaborate patterns" are essential for "memory foundation and encoding information," and it makes sense that this knowledge is immediately applicable in the classroom and lecture hall (especially for young brains that are still developing). This really resonates with me: there's something deliciously tangible about the texture of the paper, the weight of a pen in your hand, and the unique-to-you handwriting that flows onto the page; no wonder our brains light up!

## When to Do It

For almost everyone, mornings are best. You'll need just two minutes after Daily Practice #1 through #3—breathwork, stretching, and your ten minutes of challenging movement—and showering. Your Do The Thing list will certainly help structure your day, but there are no hard-and-fast rules about when you do it. Just doing it is crucial, regardless of when.

Typically, I will start to make a mental to-do list the night before when I'm stretching and breathing and thinking about the things I feel grateful for (more on that later). But what I'm really doing is getting all those worries out of my head. The next morning, after breathwork, stretching, and my maximum-effort workout, I write down my three things, then my two bonus things, and my final, rock star–worthy sixth task.

## What to Put on Your List

With your clean page in front of you, take a moment to think about what you truly want to accomplish in your life. It seems so obvious, but so many of the women I work with wonder about this very thing. I get it: our ultimate goals in life can seem hidden behind the endless noise and distraction of our daily lives and responsibilities.

In this situation, I usually turn to the Japanese concept of ikigai, the idea that finding your sense of purpose can lead to a long and happy life. There is nothing like feeling aligned with what you are doing. You might never get to that perfect alignment, or if you do, it might only be for a short while, but spending a lifetime in pursuit of it sure is a life worth living. If what you're good at, what you're passionate about, what is needed in the world, and what you can make your profession all converge into one thing, then you've achieved ikigai.

So, what is it you truly want? To riff on that question, I usually ask the following: If I had a magic wand (I imagine mine like Glinda's in *The Wizard of Oz* and *Wicked*) and was able to instantly give you one thing in your life, one achievement, what would it be? Within a few moments, most of us can come up with something specific. It usually has something to do with work or study, improving one's health (like finishing a fitness program), or setting up a dream business, rather than a tangible object like a shiny new car or a Birkin bag.

And so, I ask you now: What is the thing you most want to accomplish in life?

Perhaps you have an idea for a small business, or even a big one, but it feels like a distant dream, a cats-on-roller-skates idea that would otherwise never get off the ground. But let's really go there: What would be your very first few steps in achieving this aim?

Because I adore sweet things and go absolutely nowhere without a little treat in my handbag, let's imagine you want to open a bakery. In this fantasy, there are delicious pistachio and dark chocolate croissants displayed on vintage marble boards, a wild strawberry galette topped with rose petals, whatever your version of the cronut is, and clouds of steam from your imported Italian espresso machine—and a line out the door, of course. So, how do you Do The Thing and start the journey to realizing your bakery dream?

Have you done any research? Looked at real estate? Have you analyzed the business side of things? Have you talked to somebody who owns a bakery? Perhaps you could visit four or five successful bakehouses in nearby neighborhoods, sample their most popular products, and ask to meet with the owner, following up with a thank-you email? All small business dreams that turn into a big success started with small but significant first steps just like the ones you're now adding to your Do The Thing list.

There is another reason why it's important to take these first few steps: sometimes following your dreams means taking an unexpected turn, and that's a good thing, even if it's painful at the time. Because—and this is sometimes hard to hear—you might not actually want to open that bakery, and because you've never done the work to discover if it's something you can bring to fruition, you just dream about it your whole life. Every time you wistfully bite into that perfect pastel de nata, you'll think, *Why didn't I open that bakery?* But if you did the thing, researched the market, and talked to bakers who are losing their shirt and telling you it's the toughest industry in the world, you might think, *Oh, hell no! This isn't for me!*

And so, sometimes, Doing The Thing ends up with you letting go of a dream. It can hurt, but ultimately it's transformative. Has everything I've tried worked out? Nope. But discovering that some ideas aren't going to work, or that some roads are dead ends, is such a useful life lesson. It means you can redirect your energy and make another dream flourish. You won't regret #DTT, I promise.

## Breaking Things Down into Tasks

Once you've been really honest with yourself and identified your long- and short-term goals, break each one down into a series of tasks. Then identify those specific tasks that can be achieved that day. What do you actually need to do to feel better and to progress in the areas you need to progress? Pick three strong contenders right now.

These are your nonnegotiables.

Three tasks you will absolutely, 100 percent achieve today.

Perhaps it's paperwork that you need to read through and signed. Or scheduling a phone call with somebody you haven't talked to in a long time. That call that's overdue to a friend is something many of the women I work with (and Theo) find most challenging—it feels harder with every day that passes. Or, instead of just talking about going out, your nonnegotiable could be to schedule to meet that friend, in real life—and stick to it (if my friends are reading this, Pilates and matcha?).

Each item can be as simple as buying puppy food. It is more important that your tasks be achievable—and that they make you feel more confident—than that they be ambitious, because fulfilling your biggest ambitions takes time and patience. On one recent day, I finally took care of a stack of cardboard boxes that had accumulated in the hall. The job had been deprioritized so often, I felt like I had run a marathon when I was done!

A quick note on adding small things to your nonnegotiables, like laundry, cleaning out your refrigerator, or organizing your recycling: we might not think something so insignificant could make us happy or give movement or rhythm to our days. We might like to think only those very big life moments, like graduation or getting your dream job, can really move the needle. But those small actions add up! They're meaningful, too! Not every single thing on your to-do list needs to be a significant step toward your ultimate dream goal—you can add in a few smaller things, too.

Which brings me again to "mom guilt." Like every one of the daily practices, #DTT is about giving yourself the time and attention you deserve. It is easy to feel overwhelmed with requests from others, and setting boundaries may require a serious mindset shift. Even in 2025, women are all too often supposed to be the "best" moms, wives, employees, home cooks, housekeepers, and entertainers all at once—and to look good and super sexy while doing it. Apart from this being an incredibly gendered expectation of what a perfect parent is, I want women to give themselves permission to focus more on looking after themselves.

That's why setting boundaries with family, friends, and challenging some of those sexist expectations is integral to a happy, purposeful life for you and your loved ones. You're allowed self-care. You're allowed to grow. And you're allowed to pursue your own goals and interests, guilt-free. Some of the women I meet through my work worry about their purpose outside of being a wife or mother—I really don't want that for them, nor for me or my girls.

As women, stepping outside of the role society has written for us—even for a moment—can lead to a little unease and a lot of questions. For instance, because I travel with my work, I'm sometimes away from my girls, and people ask me all the time how I deal with mom guilt (although I've personally never heard of anyone clutching their pearls about "dad guilt"—is it even a thing?). Honestly? I don't dwell on it. I do the very best I can, which means showing up for myself and the people I love with full-out effort. I am not ashamed to dedicate time to myself every day—even if it ends up being just a few minutes.

Am I missing a kid's performance next week because I am on an important business trip? Yes. Is it going to derail who my children turn out to be as human beings? No. I'm always there when I can be, and they know that I love them. I learned early in my kids' lives that it's not my job to be at their beck and call 24/7. My job is to be sure they feel my love and support always, and I can do so while creating a business I'm proud of, something that gives the whole household the best life possible (and yes, that also goes for Chedi, our endlessly spoiled pup). To make sure I'm living the life I deserve to live, I set clear boundaries.

That said, my girls know that once I've finished with what I need to get done during the day, I'm 100 percent present. No scrolling through social media, no email. When they have me, they really have me—and I love that. But if I still have work to get done during the day, they know how to keep themselves entertained. (Just ask Lin-Manuel Miranda: boredom begets creativity! Growing up, Lin's parents worked tirelessly and, as they were often out of the house, he had to entertain himself after school. He found there is nothing better to spark creativity than time alone.) This balance means I show up for myself and everyone else in my life. And isn't that what it's all about?

## Building Your Own #DTT List

As I noted earlier, each day I write down three nonnegotiable tasks, two bonus tasks, and a feel-good activity to look forward to.

Remember that items #4 and #5 on your list are meant to be a stretch. You may not get to them right away, no matter how hard you try, and that is completely okay. They can always be #1 and #2 tomorrow.

One recent list of mine looks like this:

1. Write for two hours.
2. Clean out my junk drawer.
3. Film a workout for social media.

---

4. Drop off boxes at UPS.

5. Call my mentor for some advice.
   _____

6. Buy the girls new school socks.

When you deconstruct your to-do list and then reconstruct it in this way, it makes it so much more attainable and takes away the feeling of being overwhelmed. To rephrase: take things off your list, have a rethink, and then write down your three most important, life-moving things to do . . . and simply do them! If you can do more, that's great. But you're winning if you just do those three, because if you do those three, then things move on. They just do. You've Done The Thing. Well done, you!

Then, tomorrow, you might start with those tasks in your #4 and #5 slots, adding them as your new nonnegotiables—or create a whole new list. Overall, the radical #DTT idea is that doing less means you end up doing a little more.

Another important point: you have to be very cognizant of what you're adding to your #DTT list, and brutally honest with yourself. Don't write down what you know you can't achieve. These tasks are nonnegotiable, so if you're going to write down "go for a two-hour run" and you know you're not really going to have time for that, then don't set yourself up for failure. Ultimately, you are setting your own terms, so give yourself the best shot.

In hindsight, #DTT is taken right out of my dance training. When you are learning a dance, you simplify a complex routine by separating it into manageable small steps. You start with the first eight counts and practice the moves until you have them down pat. Then you can add on more choreography and learn the more ambitious parts of the dance that looked impossible when you started out.

It is a remarkable model for improvement—but progress feels incremental at first. You may even feel silly doing the same easy step over and over again just to commit it to muscle memory. I promise you, though: if you stick with it, you will realize it is the surest, fastest route to radical change. Consistency plus a little effort and time always delivers. And, like Sarah in chapter 3 and the mini goals that allowed her to rock-hop to fitness success, there's just no feeling like knowing you did what you set out to do.

In a 2011 study, psychologists E. J. Masicampo and Roy Baumeister at Florida State University tested out this same mini goal approach. They found that study participants who were allowed to write down an upcoming task and identify a step-by-step plan to achieve it were less anxious about it. Doing so gave them more focus and increased their chances of success. Achieving their ultimate goal became a series of smaller achievements—and each one in turn gave participants a sense of satisfaction that would otherwise have been denied to them until the grand finale. Also, knowing they were on the right track gave Masicampo's and Baumeister's subjects more bandwidth to focus on other pursuits. I believe it: I never could have built up Xtend Barre the way I did—little by little, each and every day—without #DTT.

## Adjusting Our Expectations

Of course, not everything works out the way it should, and the trail we take through life can have its pitfalls. Sometimes we must adjust our expectations, take a different route, and keep on keeping on. My friend Rockell knows all about that.

A few years ago, as I expanded Xtend Barre from my tiny guest room headquarters, it was Rockell (or, as I call her, Rocky) who encouraged me to dream big and have a truly global vision. After years dancing across the globe (hello, Moulin Rouge in Paris) and practicing Pilates, Rockell had decided to settle down a bit and open her own Pilates studios in Las Vegas. She loved Pilates and movement as much as I did, and she eventually became my international franchise partner in Australia and across the world.

From the moment we connected, I knew we were going to be friends. Rockell's whole life is built on movement, from dance to Pilates, and she's also an award-winning equestrian and showjumper, and a major horse lover. She's energetic and enthusiastic, one of those awesome women who moves through life at supersonic speed.

But shortly after I started writing this book, Rockell was in a terrible riding accident. She was thrown from her horse and couldn't move her body in the first few minutes after the accident. Airlifted to a nearby hospital on Australia's Sunshine Coast, she wasn't sure she would ever be able to move her body in the same way again. Thank goodness her sensation started to return in the hospital, and within a few days, Rockell was able to stand and even walk a few steps—but that was it. Since then, she told me, she's had to relearn how to do everything while wearing a neck brace, carefully strengthening her neck and back. As I write this, Rockell is still making headway and her progress is amazing, but it's been tough, she says. And yet, here she is, back on the trail, accepting that it's going to take longer and with smaller moves than she would like, but she'll get there.

She is taking the smallest, most challenging steps of her life at a speed she would not have chosen, so she can get back to moving artfully and elegantly through this world. That girl really is beauty in motion.

## What Happens If You *Don't* Do The Thing

We've explored how feeling overwhelmed with too many to-dos can cause us to get stuck, and how chronic procrastination can self-perpetuate, locking us into a cycle of nonachievement and even bad health outcomes. In other words, sometimes you just don't Do The Thing. Let's say, life happens, and you have to go pick up your kids from school and just don't have the time you thought you had. Give yourself some grace and step back on the wagon tomorrow (don't build that campsite!).

Still don't think you can Do The Thing? #DTT is my tried-and-tested, surefire system of getting shit done; it really works, and there's not a simpler hack out there. You're literally lowering your daily expectations and making your achievements more attainable, and from there your motivation to do more and more can only grow. Yes, #DTT might be particularly challenging for some of us, so do get evaluated if you feel you need to. A diagnosis could, in turn, reveal smart strategies that will help you soar or lead to work with a specialized coach to get the most out of your skill set. Otherwise, there is an expectation of personal responsibility with #DTT: If you don't think or don't want to Do The Thing, that's fine, but you're going to stay right where you are, honey. You're going to stay there complaining about whatever you're complaining about, feeling the way you're going to feel, and nothing's going to change. Or you could just Do The Thing and slowly, step by step, day by day, transform your life.

## . . . and What Happens If You Do

With that in mind, I should tell you about a slow burn success of mine: something that took a decade to come together. As I write this book, the Xtend Barre method I created is live over at BODi.com, a leading US health and wellness platform for celebrity trainers and instructors, with hundreds of incredible on-demand classes. It's the kind of site that became a fitness go-to during the pandemic, and I'm so proud of my content, especially as my classes have been streamed millions of times.

But getting there wasn't easy. In fact, it wasn't love at first sight between BODi and me, much to my disappointment at the time! When I first approached them, I was in my twenties, and I had the idea of making my own fitness DVD. I was young, but I knew I had incredible experience, and my confidence had grown through the countless small steps I had taken performing since I was a child. I already felt comfortable onstage, and I was sure I could present to the camera, too. To me, making a fitness DVD with BODi (known then as BeachBody) was about the coolest thing I could imagine. I knew I would be an asset to them, if only they could see it, too.

None of this seemed to make sense to BODi: they said no to me so many times. There were countless snags and unseen setbacks. In fact, it took me ten whole years to realize my dream. Year one: I went to Target with my notebook, headed straight for the fitness DVDs, and copied down the names of all the production companies. Then I went to work searching online for the right contacts, sent out my pitch emails, and received several "thanks, but no thanks" replies. I was crushed, but my desire was so strong, I dusted myself off and decided on a plan: a series of—you guessed it—small steps to Do The Thing.

Eventually, through my perseverance, I got a callback. I still remember the day I heard from a production company (not BODi) who decided to give me—this Midwestern woman they didn't know at all, but who called and emailed endlessly—a chance. They asked me to mail them a video and, much like the ballet video my dad filmed, I recorded it that same day and got it to them the next morning. Soon, they wrote me back and finally

## DO THE THING

said what I'd been waiting to hear: "Okay, you're great. We love this. We're gonna put you in touch with our best director for a film test."

Andrea Ambandos wasn't just that production company's best director; she was the best director in the industry, and she was (is) as formidable as she is talented. In other words, she's one tough cookie, and naturally she wondered what the heck she was doing with a newbie like me. "You mean to say you've never filmed fitness before?" she asked on our first get-to-know-you call, "and you have no experience whatsoever? None?" She was clearly skeptical about the project. I had to really breathe through that one. "I have no idea why they hired you," she thought out loud. "You'd better be good."

If you've seen *The Devil Wears Prada*, you'll understand the dynamics (I'm Anne Hathaway's character, just to be clear), so I made sure I wasn't just ready for the big shoot; I was overprepared. I rehearsed so many times that I knocked it out of the park on that day, I made my director very happy, and I was buzzing with excitement for what was to come.

We laugh about it now, because Andrea and I grew to adore each other; we have worked together many times, and we're close friends to this day. I'd made it. I realized one of my dreams through a series of small steps, consistency, and effort over time.

But I still hadn't made it to BODi. I reached out to them again, and now that I had a little more experience under my dance belt, I connected with Lara Ross, a producer (and now, another great friend). I let it be known that I would love to do a project with them. They were making and marketing their own fitness DVDs—for fitness nerds, their roster included P90X and Shaun T's Insanity, both now huge brands in the industry—and I wanted in!

Of course, they (very politely) pushed back. Barre, my specialty, just wasn't their thing, they explained. But little did they know that this hadn't stopped me before. I added "Call Lara" to my planner, every six months, and that's just what I did. For four years. Small steps, very slow progress, but I got there!

Lara commissioned me to run a test group featuring my barre workout and a three-month healthy eating plan to help some wonderful ladies achieve their fitness goals. But there was a snag: I was five months pregnant with my second daughter, I had some annoying temporary medical issues that meant I couldn't teach like I normally would, and the shoot would be in Los Angeles, not in Florida, where I was living. And yet, somehow, I made it work, and those ladies—well, those before-and-after shots were amazing.

But, as I had already learned, not everything happens the way you hoped it would. Although the test group was a success, the production schedule changed, things were delayed, and, in the meantime, my life began to change. My second daughter was born, and I loved being a mom again. Then, I focused on expanding my business, Xtend Barre, to grow internationally. It seemed people outside of the US really liked it! Soon, I had

XB studios across the globe. But almost at the same time, my marriage broke down.

I was an international business owner and a full-time mom to two young girls; those small steps were getting harder and harder to take. Still, I kept up my twice-yearly calls to Lara, and in 2019 it finally happened: "Are you ready to create an amazing workout program for us?"

I will never, ever forget sitting in the school parking lot waiting to pick up my girls when I heard those words. Ten years after our first conversation, I finally found my way onto BODi as a super trainer. Countless small steps later, each one getting me closer and closer to my goal, and I'd made it!

## Doing Less to Do More

Doing less to do more also helped inspire the Pomodoro Technique, the hugely popular time-management system designed by software supremo Francesco Cirillo when he was a student in the late 1980s and inspired—in part—by his cute kitchen timer shaped like a tomato. I love how the system acknowledges our mind's natural desire to wander and become distracted, especially when we're anxious or have too many to-dos. Instead of fighting this urge, the Pomodoro Technique harnesses it and uses it to help you achieve more.

Studying for an exam, Francesco just couldn't concentrate, and he found himself making a bet against time: Could he read for just two minutes until his pomodoro kitchen timer rang? He nailed it, of course! Experimenting with different periods of time, he found that studying for a series of shorter periods meant he did more overall, and the Goldilocks duration was twenty-five minutes of tough study followed by a mandatory five-minute break before starting the clock again. I'm here for anything that means you're up and away from your desk every twenty minutes or so; it's essential for your mobility and longevity. Motion is lotion, after all.

There you have it: Daily Practice #4 is a distilled to-do list with less pain and pressure, more focus, and built-in rewards, and it's immune to the effects of procrastination. Each nonnegotiable item creates a path to our ultimate dream goals, broken down into tasks that turn out to be achievable steps to ikigai greatness.

From this perspective, #DTT becomes deeply meaningful—essential, even. Your daily achievements, anything from purchasing puppy food to taking the first steps in creating a new business, form part of a larger plan to explore your purpose and create a life worth living for you and the ones you love. These small daily moves, done with consistency, full-out effort, and time, can only add up, and before you know it, you've created a big life.

Now, let's Do The Thing.

## daily practice #5

# set the table

*eating mindfully,
with pleasure, gratitude,
and (maybe) matcha*

> **WHAT WILL I BE DOING?**
> Eating your first meal of the day, mindfully.
>
> **HOW LONG WILL IT TAKE?**
> 10 minutes.
>
> **WHEN DO I DO IT?**
> Almost always in the morning or whenever you have your first meal. Oh, and we're taking a breakfast time-out, so no screens allowed.
>
> **AND WHAT WILL I ACHIEVE?**
> Presence, pleasure, and a healthy relationship with food. Girl, do you want to transform the way you eat? Silence your phone. Sit down and be present: it's just you, your breakfast, and a cup of coffee (or, in my case, matcha). It's as simple as that. Does "no screens" sound like the most challenging daily practice yet? Just wait until you hear about my "fridgervention."

I believe passionately in showing up for life's small pleasures. But Daily Practice #5 was inspired, in part, by a small pleasure I failed to enjoy. Once, years ago, I splurged for an extra ten-minute foot massage at my local nail salon. I'm not one of those girls who loves getting their nails done, but I do love a massage. It had been a long day, and I knew it would feel fantastic—but I ended up spending the whole time on my phone. A friend sent me a fun text, which started a whole conversation, GIFs were swapped, and I did not realize the massage had even started until suddenly it was over, and I was out the door in a daze.

Intellectually, I knew it had happened, but my mind had no connection to it, and therefore I just didn't feel it. The whole thing gave me such a strong sense of unease: If I couldn't even show up for the small luxury of a foot massage, what else was I missing? It was a surprisingly loud wake-up call!

In the future, I resolved not to miss a single moment and vowed never to make this mistake again—and it was not only foot massages that fell under this new rule. Although it's still a challenge sometimes to completely switch off my attention from my phone or computer (especially as social media is essential to my work, as it is for many of us), I am now so much more conscientious about what I am doing—and I get so much more from it, whether I am taking a walk with my daughters and our dog or organizing my workspace.

Most game-changing of all, for me, was how screen-free intervals changed my approach to mealtimes, especially breakfast. Daily Practice #5 came out of my growing self-awareness that every morning, while I made a sit-down meal for the kids, I always ate mine on the fly, standing at the countertop, quickly shoving in whatever food was left on my girls' plates while simultaneously going through my mental checklist for the day and making sure the girls had everything ready before heading off to school.

I was a multitasking breakfast champ, but I started to see that this was not the best way to start my day. I was really missing out, both in terms of spending time with my girls and preparing for my day. Besides, as I ate breakfast at light speed, I wasn't truly enjoying or savoring my food (heck, I often couldn't even remember what I had for breakfast). I wasn't doing a single thing intentionally.

At first, the switch-up was a challenge. As I was building my business, and because I like to do a few things at the same time, meals and snacks were always rushed. There is something to be said for that hustle mindset, but I would eat at my screen most days, completely distracted between work emails and chores, and occasionally I would even wonder: Did I eat lunch? *Girl, this is not good*, I thought.

I had to try to be more present. My kids would realize what was going on sooner than I would. "Mom, sit down," they would gently scold, and I would nod along; I had every intention of doing so once I'd finished this extremely important, just-can't-wait thing I was doing, like reorganizing the refrigerator or wiping away toast crumbs. Again, they'd say, "Mom, sit down!" and finally I would snap out of it. Now, I'm happy to say it's a habit. This might be news to some, but sitting down for breakfast at home—solo or with others—and taking a breath can be a pleasurable experience. It's even associated with improved physical and mental well-being. So, for Daily Practice #5, please join me in doing the same, each and every day: a breakfast club, if you will.

## SET THE TABLE

So, what's the first rule of breakfast club? While I now take all my meals seriously, none has proven so important to me as the first meal of the day. After I have finished my morning workout and made my #DTT list, I make sure to sit down and fuel up. Perhaps, right now, you're a count-your-calories-and-wolf-it-down kinda girl, and that's fine, but I know there's a better way.

Sitting down for ten minutes—an incredibly brief amount of time for a meal, truth be told—and mindfully eating healthy food without distraction (and yes, that means no screens and scrolling) is a mental and physical reset. When you allow yourself to really savor your food, what was once a tiny moment lost in the gaps of your day is truly elevated. Your mind will quiet and focus clearly on the day ahead; your body will be consciously satisfied, sending an essential message to your brain that you're full; you'll connect with your roommates, your partner, your kids, or just yourself; and you'll actually enjoy the experience.

And so, your goal for Daily Practice #5 is to Set the Table and sit down for a healthy breakfast for at least ten minutes.

The thinking around this is that if you do that one thing in the morning, just like if you spend a moment doing breathwork, stretching, and a mini-workout first thing, you're going to be more likely to make healthy decisions throughout the rest of your waking hours. You're not just setting the table; you're setting yourself up for a healthy day.

It doesn't need to be a marathon, and the meal doesn't have to be a big production—but if you take less time than ten minutes, you will likely be eating too quickly (and not chewing enough) to get all the nutritional goodness out of your meal and—just as important—you'll be going too fast to enjoy your food. Remember, pleasure is an essential requirement.

## The Importance of Breakfast

For this book, I reached out to the supersmart nutritionist Keri Glassman. She's my favorite healthy eating expert; you'll know her from *The Today Show*, *Good Morning America*, or her best-selling nutrition books. Plus, she's just an all-around great girl, and I wanted her take on all this.

One of the things I love about Keri's approach is that she's a realist. She really understands our relationship to food, what new habits we're likely to adopt, what we'll struggle with, and how to set her clients up for success. So much of her work is about encouraging us to "eat empowered," and I'm all for it.

As I suspected, for Keri breakfast is nonnegotiable. "That first meal is crucial," Keri told me. "There are many, many, many reasons why you need breakfast, whatever time of the day you have it, from helping stabilize your blood sugar throughout the morning to providing satiety throughout the day, cognitive performance, even setting up healthy habits later on.

"But this idea of sitting down for breakfast and setting the tone, it's like when I tell people to start the day with a glass of water with lemon: there's a mental component to it," she explained. "Aside from the fact that you're adding to your hydration for the day, you're doing something that's mentally good for you." She referenced onetime Navy SEAL William H. McRaven's amazing book *Make Your Bed*, which is all about celebrating the "small victories" in our daily lives. "There's a symbolic, psychological aspect to it," she said, "and there's a physiological aspect to it, too.

"There are three things going on here. One, when you sit down for breakfast, or any meal, you're more aware of how much you're eating," said Keri. "Now, if you've served yourself a portioned amount, sitting or standing won't change the quantity, but you're going to be more mindful. Second, you're going to eat slower, and that helps you feel fuller; you're just more satisfied versus eating something as you're walking through the kitchen or unloading the dishwasher, when you don't really feel like you've had a proper meal." I think I instinctively bit my lip when Keri said that—it absolutely used to be me! "And third, when you're more relaxed before you eat, your digestive tract is in a place to absorb nutrients better. There is a benefit to being in that calmer state."

In *The Mind-Gut Connection*, Emeran Mayer's bestselling book, Mayer says that just as we look at someone and can tell they are scared or angry, it's the same with their gut. Keri explained, "If you knew what those signs were—and he gives examples in the book—you could tell how someone feels by looking at their gut. It's really freaking cool!" That means if you're anxious and nervous, "your gut is not in a place to absorb your nutrients as well. But if you're calm, not only do you eat slower, but you also chew your food better, break it down better, and your gut is going to be able to digest better."

Considering how important breakfast is, I asked Keri how she helps clients who struggle to really nail that first meal of the day. "One thing I always tell people is, if you have a really tough time with breakfast, have a simple alternative you can easily rotate to, one you always have the ingredients for," she said. "That way, if you get sick of one dish, there's another one. It's not complicated, and you don't have to go to the grocery store for a million things. Just concentrate on two meals you love. It might be eggs and spinach on sprouted grain toast, or yogurt and berries and chia seeds—just always have those few items in the house."

This idea makes great sense to me, as I eat pretty much the same every single day. Not being the best chef in the world (my girls will surely agree with that take), I love to repeat the recipes I'm good at and make sure I always have those ingredients in the house. You might be more adventurous, but for me, it makes for an easy-to-put-together breakfast I know I'm going to love.

## Please Sit Down

Every one of my daily practices is about self-care, and breakfast time is no different. As you would with a foot massage, you should be able to focus completely on what you're doing. I know many, many women think they must "fit in" meals, especially breakfast and lunch, between their daily tasks. They might even eat breakfast on the move as they are getting the kids ready for school or driving to work. This is all wrong—you need this time for yourself! Take it seriously, enjoy your food, and sit down at the kitchen table.

Studies show differences in how quickly you digest your food depending on whether you're standing, sitting, or lying down. Due to the risk of indigestion or even choking, the latter isn't generally advised (although that doesn't stop me from munching on popcorn while lying on the couch with my girls for movie night), but standing or sitting have similar physical effects.

What's fascinating to me is the admittedly small area of research around our enjoyment of food and how our seating options might play a part. To share a story I came across when researching this chapter, it seems sitting down might make what you're eating seem even tastier. Professor Dipayan Biswas, a "sensory marketing expert" at the University of South Florida Muma College of Business, authored a study in which participants enjoyed the same snack (a pita chip) far more when seated in a comfortable chair, and failed to notice that brownie squares from a local restaurant had been secretly spiked with too much salt when the testers were standing uncomfortably. This is good enough for me! Sit down, give yourself a moment, and your food awareness will grow, and whatever is on your plate might just taste better, too.

Good posture—and that means feet flat on the floor, knees level with your hips, shoulders relaxed—during mealtime will minimize post-meal reflux and aid healthy digestion. By being mindful, you will also be able to tell more quickly when you have reached satiety and when you are just eating to eat. Besides all the other reasons to correct your posture, this is a huge benefit for your health.

I'm not asking you to eat every single meal sitting down, and I'm not asking you to do everything perfectly. But I want you to sit down and give yourself just ten uninterrupted minutes for that first meal of the day. Whether you eat it at six in the morning or you eat it at noon, put your phone away, be present with your kids, your partner, your cat, whoever's next to you, or just be present with yourself.

## Matcha Mindfulness

Guess who has a matcha obsession and isn't afraid to admit it? This girl! Apart from being completely delicious, adding matcha to my breakfast routine has taught me a few things. I know this seems like "matcha do about nothing" (I'm here all week!), but hear me out. This mysterious potion is made from green tea leaves milled into a soft, fine powder and then whisked with hot water or milk to make a revitalizing drink that has the creamy texture of a latte, and I happen to absolutely love it.

The production process is so thoughtful and intricate: tea bushes are grown in the shade, and just after harvesting, the young leaves are steamed (to retain their bright green tone) and then baked before being cut, dried again, and stone-milled to create a powder. You can use a special ceramic measuring spoon, a tiny fine-net tea strainer to sift the matcha, and, after adding just-boiled filtered water, a Chasen, the traditional bamboo tea whisk, to briskly stir up the infusion until it has a fine, textured foam. Even with the instant matcha I love, there is no other way to make this delicious drink than doing it slowly and methodically; there's an art to it! And then there's that first sip, the subtle bitterness, nutty sweetness, and that soft umami note; it tastes so vibrantly green. I love that first sip of green goodness; it truly feels like a mini spa moment for me.

Why am I telling you all this? Good question. The process of making matcha—and remembering its journey to your cup each morning—can only be a mindful one. This is because it requires concentration, patience, and a little effort and skill. You become aware of your surroundings, the sensations of warm steam, the fragrant aroma, and the weight of the cup or bowl in your hand; the whole experience is a mini lesson in being in the moment. That's what I really need in the mornings—plus, it tastes great, too!

In terms of using awareness as a route to pleasure, ancient Greek philosopher Epicurus, influential author of around three hundred treatises, is a good reference point here. While other great thinkers of his era were focused on the meaning of existence, Epicurus just wanted to be happy, and thought this could be achieved not by the pursuit of romance, status, or luxury, but through the pleasure of simplicity, eating well, and—I'm paraphrasing here—living in the moment. If being Epicurean means being mindful and allowing yourself a moment to enjoy daily life and feel a little gratitude for its simplest pleasures, then I'm with the ancient guy with the beard.

## Start the Day Phone-Free

Setting the table, and setting ourselves up for success, can only happen if we're truly focused. That means putting down our phones. This, I know, is harder than it seems. Social media algorithms that personalize our digital experiences are incredibly sophisticated and intuitive, offering an endless scroll of information and entertainment. Wait, do I need to buy that? Did that dog just say "I love you"? It's weird but addictive. But we all know that too much screen time can make us lose focus, distract us from what we need to do, and lock us in a sad cycle of half-achievements that leave us feeling inadequate and burnt out.

That's why a no-screens rule at breakfast is essential. Daily Practice #5, Set the Table, is not just a ten-minute exercise in nutrition, it's also a rare interlude in which to clear your mind and focus on the real world: the sensory pleasures of great food, the calming peace to think and plan uninterrupted, and the opportunity to connect with your loved ones. If we truly want to examine our potential, achieve our goals, be more productive and engaged, and experience (and remember) pleasure, then we must relearn how to focus.

Research suggests that, for today's students at least, smartphones aren't making anyone smarter. In fact, there is some evidence that suggests young people are becoming less intellectually sharp and finding it hard to forge strong real-life friendships. High schoolers are reporting worse emotional well-being and test scores than in previous years, and in 2024, US Surgeon General Vivek H. Murthy weighed in, writing in *The New York Times* that he was issuing a "warning label on social media platforms" pointing out their negative effects on youth mental health. It follows that starting the day phone-free—just for ten minutes—creates opportunity for focus, allowing you to think through your Do The Thing goals and truly enjoy your meal.

## The Whole Story: What to Eat

More than anything else, what makes a meal healthy is the presence of whole foods. You know what I mean: unprocessed, unadulterated, un-messed-around-with, and almost always market fresh. As tempting as processed foods may be, resist them—at least for breakfast. They might be convenient, but they aren't nutrient-dense; they're low in fiber and high in sodium; and they're hard to digest.

What's more, processed foods just don't satisfy: you'll be running on empty before you know it, and when your blood sugar levels are low, your stomach secretes ghrelin, a hormone that tells your brain you need to eat. This stimulates your appetite, making you hungry again too soon.

But if you aim for protein, whole grains, veggies, and healthy fats in your breakfast, you're golden. By "healthy fats," I'm talking about what you get from whole foods like eggs and avocado. (Side note: slicing avocado always makes me think of Scott Metzger's Avocado Affirmation cartoon—you know the one; it's been memed a thousand times—where a plump avocado stands "naked" in front of a bathroom mirror, affirming himself with the words "You're fat, but you're *good* fat.") Follow this rule and you'll be pleasantly full and energized for hours.

"It can absolutely take some work," says Keri, "but if you can get to a place where you're eating until you're slightly satisfied, eating when you're slightly hungry, and eating whole, real foods for the most part, then you're never going to overeat."

This was something I already knew instinctively. Eating well, eating intentionally, and enjoying your food means your body and mind are getting what they need—and no more.

Researchers who study the science of eating rates can't seem to agree on the perfect eating speed, how long we should chew each mouthful, or if long, drawn-out mealtimes really do improve our health stats. But eating slowly—or more slowly than usual—is generally associated with healthier outcomes, and that's good enough for me. Because improving your physical health isn't the only reason I want you to take a moment over your morning meal—I want you to have the opportunity to improve your mental health and general sense of well-being, too. Join me: Set the Table.

## Organization Is Key

If you are anxious about adding a sit-down breakfast to your morning routine, if you're thinking, *How will I ever find the time?*, try rethinking how you plan your meals. Rather than opening the refrigerator and wondering what you could eat—and therefore only increasing the temptation of eating ultra-processed, ready-to-go foods—always have a few mealtime favorites.

In addition to repeating the same combinations week in, week out, Keri recommended another way to make a mindful breakfast easier: "I don't meal prep, I ingredient prep," she said. "Well, that's why we're aligned!" I replied (I have so much time for this girl—she knows her stuff!). I make sure all the healthy ingredients I need are right there for me: celery chopped for my tuna, cucumbers sliced for my salad, eggs hardboiled for my snack, watermelon sliced for dessert. I eat similar meals every morning for breakfast; I have a few rotating lunches; and I make a handful of easy dinner recipes that I absolutely love.

Maybe you are more ambitious in the kitchen than I am—all power to you!—but you don't need to go to great lengths to eat well. One key benefit of my repeatable meals is that I know how each ingredient makes me feel. If you rely on a specific set of ingredients, it is easy to recalibrate when something in your repertoire is not making you feel good.

## Stage a Fridgervention

There's one foolproof strategy I always recommend: a "fridgervention." Yes, that means it may be time to take a long, critical look inside the refrigerator and start swapping out some of the unhealthy foods you find for better options (and get rid of that six-month-old pickle jar with its one solitary pickle while you're at it!).

When you open my fridge, you'll see a variety of real foods in various colors. I invested in sturdy glass and biosafe plastic containers, so I can see every food item on the shelf (I also get a small thrill from organized spaces). This way, I can see what looks fresh, and I can keep everything extra clean. I shop a few times a week, and as soon as I arrive home from the grocery store, I cut my fruits and veggies into easy-to-grab pieces (if I say "I'll wash this later," it never gets done. Then a week later I'm looking at that moldy bowl of berries or soggy greens). I even stack eggs into a clear, open container.

When I'm done, it all looks so enticing—for a few hours, at least, until the kids dive in for snacks and wreck my Martha Stewart dreams. When healthy food looks good, you expect it to taste good, too.

## Leveling Up: Tips for Keeping Healthy Eating in Mind

Here are my tried-and-true tips for eating healthfully, even when your busy life makes you want to reach for the nearest microwave dinner.

### *80/20 Eating*

If sitting down, phone-free, for just ten minutes is the first rule of breakfast club, another important breakfast-time habit (and habit for every meal) is my 80/20 rule. Similar to Keri's recommendation to focus on eating healthfully at least eighteen out of twenty-one of your weekly meals (more on that in a moment), my 80/20 rule has been a game changer for me—it means I can be mindful of what I'm eating without necessarily counting calories or endlessly tracking macros—and even allows flexibility for treats and surprises. Here is how you do it.

## Eat Until You're 80 Percent Full

First, eat until you feel 80 percent full. That's it! When you're filling your plate, it's so easy to give yourself more than you need. In my experience, there is no benefit to eating more than that—even the taste becomes less fun. By the time you have reached 80 percent full, you are probably actually satiated, but your body needs a moment to catch up.

When we have eaten what we need, our fat tissues secrete leptin, a hormone that tells the brain we're done. It's a completely natural response, but those "Whoa, slow down!" signals from our digestive system take a beat to kick in—some research suggests it can take around twenty minutes—and we can usually eat faster than these signals are received and processed. So it makes sense that we might end up eating more than we need if we don't realize we're full until way after the fact.

We can override those feelings easily, especially if we really, really love what we're eating (like that second or third slice of peach pie at Thanksgiving). Remember, meals are not a now-or-never, this-is-your-last-chance situation. That 20 percent you're not eating does not go to waste: you'll keep whatever it is for leftovers and pick it up later, so take a few minutes after each serving to see how you feel.

When I first read about 80/20 eating, it was a real light-bulb moment, because I'd been doing it intuitively for years. Being a dancer and having a crazy training and audition schedule meant I only ever ate until I was around 80 percent full anyway. I was active, so I had a great appetite, but I never wanted to overdo it, as I would usually have to perform again a couple of hours later. That meant I was never that person who gorged at dinner to the "I need to undo my pants" point—impossible if I had to then go do kicks and leaps. To this day, I just don't like the feeling of being uncomfortably full.

Let's quickly head over to the University of Adelaide to meet researchers Monica Beshara, Amanda D. Hutchinson, and Carlene Wilson, who studied a sample of South Australians and their eating habits back in 2013. They asked participants to self-report how much they ate, focusing on serving size, and got them to compare their meals with what they ate the previous week. Perhaps being part of a research project and knowing their actions were being reviewed made the participants more conscious of their eating habits, but the study showed this mindful approach meant less food consumption overall as time went on. The participants ate a little less when they were more focused on their mealtime.

Consider this as we explore the 80/20 method's second aspect:

## Eat Healthy 80 Percent of the Time

There's no need to throw yourself into an all-or-nothing diet (or the perfectionism that comes with it). Diets may be effective in the short term, but zoom out and you'll realize they do nothing to foster long-term healthy eating, which is the real key to creating a body you love. If you eat as healthfully as possible 80 percent of the time, you will get all the nutrition you need to power your day—and you can have fun with the last 20 percent.

Of course, the aim should be to eat with pleasure 100 percent of the time, but that final 20 percent? Give yourself a break and a little love. And if that looks like cheesecake to you, well, that's fine. Personally, I adore an occasional chocolate treat!

What we choose to eat and drink doesn't just have nutritional value. It has emotional value, too. From kids' first birthday parties to late-night dinners with old school friends to lavish, upscale wedding banquets and down-home cookouts with hot dogs and s'mores, food is forever linked to life's most important and memorable moments. Meals and snacks punctuate our days, adding interludes, quick moments of connection, or a welcome full stop at the end of a busy week, just like how that perfectly stirred, ice-cold martini served in a chilled vintage coupe on a Friday evening tells you that work has ended (oh, how I love a chilled glass!) and the weekend has begun. We owe it to ourselves to consciously experience the pleasures these moments offer.

## Zooming Out

I asked Keri about that guilty feeling around eating something "bad." We might try our best to eat healthfully all week, but then we slip up, lick the ketchup from our fingers, and feel awful about it. "People get thrown off if they have just one totally indulgent meal," said Keri. "Maybe it was out of their control, they might be at a dinner party and it's the only thing being served, or maybe they just really craved it; they were having a bad day and ate a big portion of fries and fried chicken and whatever. Everybody has those emotional situations sometimes, and you can't beat yourself up for that either."

Keri has a clever solution to make sure her clients aren't being too hard on themselves: "Aim for eighteen out of twenty-one intentional meals a week," she said. "That way you can still make a few conscious indulgences and know you're totally hitting your target." Here, Keri is asking us to zoom out so we can see the bigger picture: a week of mainly healthy, delicious meals means the odd pleasure-only snack is totally allowed. So, you ate some mozzarella sticks: Who cares?

## *Trying to Lose Weight? What Can you Eat More Of?*

Another reason I love eating like this is that I have always tended to push back on traditional diet advice. Instead, I want to maintain a set of uncomplicated habits for mindful eating and a nutritious menu. I'm not a fan of diets that are too restrictive or cutting calories so drastically that you're left feeling weak, irritable, and trying to ignore your hunger pangs. Food deprivation is never, ever effective long term. While it might make you temporarily lighter, it will steal your energy and compromise your muscle mass. Nor do I want anyone to force down low-cal meals that are beige and boring—I definitely wouldn't do this myself. Life's too short!

Perhaps you want to tone up, increase your stamina, or lose a little weight and up your health stats along the way? There's one question I like to ask here, and it's usually met with a *WTF?* response.

Here goes: What can you add to your daily diet to help you achieve this?

I just love how counterintuitive this sounds. Shouldn't we be removing things from our menu, not adding them? Well, nope, not if you're eating whole foods with lots of protein, fiber, and good fats. If we become a little more conscious of our food choices, prepare well, and eat mindfully, we can transform our relationship with our diet—and eat with pleasure.

## Focusing on the Aftereffect

When I was about twelve or thirteen years old and dancing was my life, I entered a competition called Dupree. It was the go-to regional dance competition throughout the United States, and I was so pumped! One thing about Dupree is that, as exciting as it is, it's also challenging: you participate in classes all day long from sunrise until sunset and then compete in the evenings.

## SET THE TABLE

It's quite a task in terms of endurance, and you're also trying to impress teachers who are going to be your judges later that night. In each class, you want them to see you and notice you—you have to be full-out.

After a successful morning, I had lunch with all my dance girlfriends, my mom, and all her mom friends, too (dance moms really turn up for their kids), and I ordered a cola. I wasn't really allowed to be a big soda drinker as a kid, but I felt like I needed that surge of sugar to give me a little jolt of energy to get me through the rest of the day. Within minutes, I felt great, and I was buzzing (think: small kid, very big soda), but half an hour later I was back in class and . . . I did not feel good, not at all. It felt like my body was moving slower, my stomach was heavier, and I was so sluggish, it was harder for me to hit those sharp movements.

It was my first real experience of a sugar high followed by a sugar crash. That cola did not sit well with my body, and I wasn't able to perform at my best. I was able to rally and still do well (dancing was my life, after all), but I learned about the aftereffect at that very young age. Some foods, especially sugary or salty snacks and soda—as delicious as they are—have an aftereffect. And, to me, those aftereffects are often not worth those few seconds of deliciousness. My Dupree sugar crash really set the tone for how I eat as an adult; it doesn't mean I never indulge in a soda or sugary snack, but if I have somewhere to be, a class to lead, or there's an event I'm chairing, I don't indulge in things that are going to make me feel less than great.

It's a simple trick. If you're craving the thing you're trying to avoid, whether it's ice cream or a bag of chips, just focus on the aftereffect. This isn't about feeling guilty or scolding yourself. It's about being honest and open about what it will do to your body: you're probably going to feel lousy afterward, and no one wants that.

This hardly matters if you have a bag of candy at the movie theater; you might feel damn good because you haven't had candy in a month and it's a fantastic, mindful, indulgent moment that you should enjoy without guilt. But if you're craving fast food French fries ahead of a busy work afternoon, presentation, or trip, then you have a decision to make. Being mindful of the aftereffects of what you're eating, drinking, and doing is a game changer.

## Combat Cravings with Healthy Alternatives

Another way forward is to work *with* your desires rather than against them. I love to snack; with this in mind, my daily ingredient prep really comes into its own. Let's say I feel like something sweet and, when I open my refrigerator, all I see is an array of delicious-looking, jewel-toned chopped fruits, from watermelon chunks and orange segments to kiwi slices, then that's just what I'll have. If I'm feeling hungry for something savory and filling, and I have already prepped some freshly boiled eggs, that's what I'll have with a little smoked sea salt and a pinch of paprika; or my favorite tuna snack on a delicious, seeded cracker, stacked with crunchy pre-chopped celery. The reverse is true, too. If my fridge is full of processed convenience foods—which I'm sure will be completely delicious in a super salty and sweet way—then that's what I'd probably have. Only it won't satisfy my hunger or nutritional needs. It's just not worth it.

Once you start Daily Practice #5 and connect with this intentional approach to morning mealtime, the same approach tends to spill out into the rest of the day and week. For instance, you'll think, *I'm going to eat a better lunch because I already know I can achieve a healthy breakfast. I don't want to mess up my day with crap.* And when you go to the store, you'll notice a change of mindset: *I'm doing this breakfast thing at the moment*, you'll think. *I'm just concentrating a bit more and prepping healthier food.* So you'll pick up more fruit and veggies than usual, or maybe some healthier bread, eggs, lox, and avocado.

## Making the Change and Committing to It

A note about making the change to healthy and mindful eating and finding it overwhelming. I talk to lots of women who have a strained relationship with food. Some of us have got it down—we know what we like, we eat well, and we allow ourselves the occasional treat (that's essential, if you ask me). But others have history here, managing it as best they can, often in a way that can only be described as "It's complicated."

I want you to give yourself the very best chance at success, and that's just what Set the Table (and all my daily practices) is designed to do. You've done your breathwork, your stretching, and your workout. You've spent two minutes of focused energy and mapped out your day, identifying three nonnegotiables to head up your #DTT list—you're already winning! Now, all I want you to do is enjoy your breakfast. That's it. I need you to sit down for ten minutes, catch your breath, and be mindful as you eat.

Perhaps eating at home is just not viable? Maybe you're a New Yorker and you usually start your day grabbing a takeout coffee and scarfing down a bagel, and off you go. Maybe you're running around at lunch, and pushing it later just isn't going to work for you. I just want you to schedule those ten minutes for mindful eating. It's a priority and sets your intention for the rest of the day. Trust me on this (and enjoy that bagel).

It doesn't matter where you are or what time it is. Daily Practice #5 just requires you to not be on your phone. To not be distracted. Try to sit and enjoy your meal—for just ten minutes. Even if you're on a park bench and Set the Table turns out to be a napkin draped over one knee and a pigeon on your shoulder, you can do this!

To be clear, this isn't about counting calories, measuring macros, or restricting your diet. It's about developing your mindset toward food and taking pleasure in the moment. Perhaps you have ambitious, long-term health or weight goals? Great! But start here, start small, be mindful, and everything else will start to fall into place.

## daily practice #6

# mind up

*rewire your brain to live
with gratitude and attitude*

> **WHAT WILL I BE DOING?**
> Recording and repeating life-shifting affirmations; it's a workout for the mind.
>
> **HOW LONG WILL IT TAKE?**
> 2 minutes, minimum.
>
> **WHEN DO I DO IT?**
> Mornings or evenings, but you can hit playback throughout the day, whenever you feel you really need to hear it.
>
> **AND WHAT WILL I ACHIEVE?**
> This daily practice will help you maintain your sense of who you are and what you believe in. It can even improve your motivation and general outlook on life just by . . . talking to yourself. I get it: it sounds weird, but the science behind this is sound. It worked for me, and with consistency, it will work for you, too!

Years ago, I talked my way out of one of the worst situations of my life. In the early days of my relationship breakdown, positive verbal affirmations—along with breathwork—became a key part of my daily survival. Slowly but surely, I let my own voice guide me out of the gloom until I found solid ground again.

At the time, it felt like life was a dumpster fire. I was in shock and desperate for anything that would help. I already had a habit of occasionally writing down my hopes and dreams, but I came across a simple app that allowed me to dictate and record my own affirmations with daily reminders to play them back. But it seemed like a long shot: Could I really pull myself out of an awful situation with a five-second practice? In the end, I persuaded myself, despite feeling quite embarrassed and even a little pathetic sitting there talking to myself *about* myself, but I just knew I had to shift my energy, and this was something I was willing to try. My first recording was far from a TED talk, but I soon realized it didn't have to sound perfect or pretty: I just had to be myself. "I'm grateful for the good in my life," I finally said into my iPhone, not really believing it could help. "I have the power to shape my ideal reality."

I reminded myself that, in the past, I had found talking out loud to encourage or congratulate myself often worked wonders. I'd always done it. In training, at auditions, and before and after life's challenging moments, big or small, I'll let out a "Girl, you did good!" under my breath. And so, if the idea of using positive verbal affirmations when I was at my lowest felt a little Live, Laugh, Love, I didn't care—back then, I would have tried anything.

For me, letting my own voice encourage me was my saving grace. During the hardest times, I listened to my affirmations at least five times a day. It was like future me had sent a message back through time, telling me just what I needed to hear. "Andrea, you know your worth, you know your value, you know you're going to get to the other side of this." And without realizing how much, man, did I need to hear it. I also needed to say it out loud to really believe it, and I needed to listen to those affirmations every time I felt like I was about to crumble and collapse on the bathroom floor.

So, what are affirmations, anyway? They are present-tense statements about yourself, audiotaped or written down. They can be scribbled on sticky notes and placed all around your home, from your bathroom mirror to the refrigerator. They also can be said out loud, recorded, and played back several times a day, which is what Daily Practice #6 is all about.

Doing this is not "manifesting" or anything to do with crystals or chakras (although if that's your thing, you go for it—no questions asked). Affirmations are rooted in brain science. In fact, if affirmations are anything, they're a workout for your mind. Just like you might target your abs, arms, or legs with repetitive movements and great form, affirmations are repeated phrases that imprint on your brain's pathways.

## Why It Works

To understand how affirmations work, we need to talk a little about neuroplasticity. When we learn something new, the brain rewires itself. New synapses, or connections between neurons, form, and everything is shuffled around and reorganized to incorporate this fresh information. This "neural coding" is how we learn and create memories, especially when we're young.

But every experience, not just the good ones, leaves its mark on the brain, and as easily as some connections are made, others are bypassed or broken. We know that stress, for example, can break these connections and inhibit the forming of new synapses, meaning our brains are less malleable and aren't working as well as they might. Put simply, happy brains are squishy ones.

As we age, our brains become a little less squishy. This explains that, while it might be challenging to learn a new language as you get older, you can instantly recall something from your youth in vivid detail, like all the lyrics to Whitney Houston's version of "I Will Always Love You" (just me?). It figures that we need to find ways to retain as much neuroplasticity as possible, or use our brains more effectively, so we can continue to learn new things, create amazing memories, and avoid depression and anxiety.

The good news is we can use our neuroplasticity to introduce and embed new ideas and new beliefs that might just pull us into the light. We don't have to be passive and allow our experiences of trauma and pain, or the disappointments of the past, to forever give shape to our brains. We can make active efforts to restructure and rebuild our thought processes and override those tired old go-to phrases that pop up when we're sad or stressed, like "I'm not good enough" or "Nothing good ever happens to me." And we can do this through positive affirmations, repeated throughout the day.

Have you ever had a dream so vivid, so lifelike, you thought it was real? Or watched a movie full of jump scares and amazing feats and felt genuinely scared, stressed, or thrilled? You *knew* none of it was truly happening, but you felt the emotion anyway—and in some ways, your brain can't tell the difference. It's the same for visualization: Simply imagine a truly stressful situation (mine would be running late for a flight—this happened recently on a trip to host my Italy retreat and I made the flight by minutes! Damn you, NYC traffic!). Your brain will light up as if you're really doing it. Now, imagine repeating the same exercise but with a positive affirmation, visualizing while you do it. On some level, your brain will think it's real and, with repetition, your optimistic thoughts will start to stick.

This theory of neuroplasticity became particularly useful when all of us—and I mean the whole world—went through the same stressful and traumatic experience at the same time. The COVID-19 pandemic meant that the number of Americans who reported symptoms of anxiety or depression soared, and in "addition to diagnosable symptoms," notes Dana Smith in the *MIT Technology Review*, "plenty of people reported experiencing pandemic brain fog, including forgetfulness, difficulty concentrating, and general fuzziness." Researchers doubled their efforts in looking for ways to un-fog the brain and use neuroplasticity to get things flowing again.

Stress, one of the pandemic's side effects, can change the structure of your brain. Those stress hormones, like cortisol—essential for your fight-or-flight response—start to have a negative effect if they are present in the body in high levels and for too long. For example, over time, cortisol might shrink the hippocampus, "which is important for both memory and mood," says Smith, pointing out that "a smaller hippocampus is one of the hallmarks of depression." In fact, "many psychologists have attributed pandemic brain fog to chronic stress's impact on the prefrontal cortex, where it can impair concentration and working memory."

## Don't Write It Down, Shout It Out!

As I devised Daily Practice #6, I had already played around with affirmations and knew something of their power. I had a beautiful journal and, almost every night, for years, I would write down what I was grateful for on the left-hand page. On the right-hand page, I wrote out my hopes and dreams, but as if they had already happened. Something like, "I'm grateful I expanded Xtend Barre into a new territory," or "I'm grateful for my girls adjusting to their new school so well." When a dream moved from the right-hand page to the left-hand one, it felt like magic.

In the process of writing this book, I went back to that old journal. In some ways, it was a tough read: I wrote it when I was still in my marriage and a few of those hopes and dreams were destined to never get off the ground. Heartbreaking, of course, but, from where I am now in my life, many of those things I wished for in that journal are the last thing I would want right now. And I don't feel sad for the woman I was back then, who had those hopes for the future. Understanding life's big events is a work in progress, and for me, accepting the ebbs and flows is enough.

But in my time of crisis, I knew I needed a new way of doing things. "Time to shake things up and try something different," I told myself. I started researching wellness strategies and read up on brain science. I discovered there is something truly powerful about hearing your own voice. As kids, we tend to verbalize almost everything, saying all our thoughts and feelings out loud in a stream of words and songs. As we grow and develop, our speech becomes more sophisticated and our thinking voice becomes an inner monologue. Your own voice's unique lineage—from inner thought to familiar sound—means it has an incredibly authentic and intimate relationship with your brain. I saw that playing back audio of my own voice could make an incredible impact. So I closed and packed away my journal and recorded my affirmations verbally, listening to them when I felt most anxious.

It was a game changer. The process of creating my affirmations, recording them in the app, helped uncover an inner voice I had all but forgotten—and I was surprised how powerful it sounded. Growing up, I was a very confident kid and would easily say to myself, "You've got this thing." These new verbal affirmations made it feel like that kid was back in the room.

I soon had a name for this positive new approach: Mind Up. Through upbeat affirmations, personal to me, recorded and played back with consistency, I was able to gain strength, optimism, and hope for the future—and if I needed to get back there quickly, to steady myself or calm my anxieties, the phrase would pop up in my head. "Andrea," I would say, no doubt startling my dog, "Mind Up."

## How to Do It

For Daily Practice #6, I want you to record your own daily affirmations and play them back every day to help reset, refocus, and perhaps even (re)discover a more confident inner voice. You'll need to be creative, curious, kind to yourself, and aware of your goals. You'll also need your phone (and later, a set of headphones), a quiet space, and just two minutes.

Ready? Let's Mind Up.

Nobody loves the sound of their own voice on tape, but there is real power in hearing it! So, first, you will need to get the heck over any embarrassment you might have.

Put any self-consciousness aside, get into a private, comfortable space, turn on "voice memos" or the audio recording app on your phone, and—here's the creative part—start talking about what you are grateful for.

I want you to record four or five affirmations.

Speak slowly, calmly, and with hope.

Try to make short statements. Focus on powerful, meaningful sentences that are personal to you.

For some of us, it's *not* easier said than done. That first session might be more of a brainstorm; perhaps you haven't thought about your life in this way before, or perhaps it feels uncomfortable to say these things out loud.

Here's a nudge: you might say something similar to "I am grateful for my kids," "I am grateful for my work," or "I am grateful for my health."

It's important to devise your own. They need to be directly applicable to you, personally. Unless you already believe what you're saying, a prepackaged affirmation just won't do.

These first few will become your gratitude affirmations.

Next, try turning your mind gently to the future—for example, "I have the power to make the life I want for myself," or "I am grateful for my thriving new business."

As you speak, close your eyes and let the positivity of your affirmations flow over you. This part might seem a little woo-woo, but there's method to the madness: If you truly believe your affirmations, your brain is more likely to embed them; they will more effective.

What does that gratitude look like to you? For me, I might picture myself hugging my girls, accepting an award, addressing thousands of people, or holding hands with the love of my life.

As you listen back, don't judge yourself—you're (probably) neither an audio engineer nor a voice actor—but give yourself the same kind of love and support you would give your family. If you're embarrassed, my hack is to close your eyes as you listen back—it really works! When I listen to my affirmations, it makes me feel like a confident, driven force, and it can do the same for you.

## Some Gratitude Affirmation Ideas

There is only space for positive self-talk when it comes to moving toward a goal. I sometimes even text a friend and say, "Today we are going to turn every single negative to a positive. Deal?" When I start to think, *This seems too daunting*, or *I am not up for this*, I stop myself right there! I counter each limiting thought: *I am fueled by the challenge. I can do this.*

For your daily practice, or for the moments when a diminishing thought just keeps breaking through, I recommend trying gratitude phrases like these to Mind Up:

> I am grateful for all the good in my life.
> I am grateful for my professional success.
> I am grateful to feel so loved by so many people.
> I am grateful for my self-confidence.
> I am grateful for my strong and capable body.
> I am grateful to be in a healthy relationship.
> I am grateful for the friendships in my life.
> I am grateful to live in a happy home.
> I am grateful for how I have grown.
> I am so proud of my consistent efforts.

Still struggling to find the perfect affirmation? Don't worry, I got you. There are more examples later in this chapter, including my own personal affirmations, ones I use with my kids, and even some smart tips from my favorite big thinkers.

## When to Do It

Replay your affirmations every day. For your first few days of Daily Practice #6, I want you to Mind Up in the evening when you're calm and almost ready to end your day, taking two whole minutes to do it.

But, as time passes, you can level up and absolutely find the time of the day that works best for you. This could be first thing in the morning, right after your breathing and stretching, but for me, the evening works best (that's when any worrisome, self-sabotaging thoughts might creep in, right?), so Daily Practice #6 is a lovely thing for me to do at night, sitting up in bed or in a space by myself. It reframes my thinking, so I can refocus and then get ready for my final Daily Practice (more on that in the next chapter).

## How to Create Effective Affirmations

Here are the things to keep in mind when crafting affirmations to make them truly effective.

## *Know That Your Voice Has Power*

So, how might saying affirmations out loud help improve our brain health? Claude M. Steele is considered the creator of affirmation theory, and his work in the late 1980s, particularly his analysis "The Psychology of Self-Affirmation," remains the main reference point for anyone interested in the science. Steele probably didn't realize his research would spark a New Age movement with countless self-help books and bestsellers about manifesting, but his core findings are simple and science-based—and I love that.

Steele's studies suggested that, when it comes to your sense of self, affirmations make you resilient. Saying or writing the things you truly believe, repeated in positive phrases, can strengthen your resolve, meaning your affirmations are like armor to protect you from daily disappointments, missteps, or snarky comments. If we really, truly believe our affirmations, then conflicting information, like negative thoughts about ourselves, will be more easily dismissed. We just won't buy it.

A 2010 study in *Clinical Psychology Review* goes even further: Optimism creates resilience. People who maintain a hopeful outlook weather adversity and achieve better social and economic results than their pessimistic peers. I knew I needed a lifeline that would pull me back to a positive outlook when I was feeling down. I needed to keep moving forward, meeting my goals (however modest), and giving myself a new narrative about who I was.

Affirmation advocate David Schechter, MD, author of *The MindBody Workbook*, uses affirmation theory with chronic pain sufferers, teaching his patients to both journal and use affirmations to soothe symptoms. "Just as we do repetitive physical exercise to get stronger," he writes in *Psychology Today*, "affirmations can be thought of as exercise for our mind/brain."

Dr. Schechter uses the "analogy of 'reprogramming' our brain," saying, "Learning to think differently is part of how we learn to get rid of the pain pathways and replace them with new circuitry." Excitingly, he even says that some data "suggests that recording the affirmation and hearing it aloud in your own voice may be more powerful than internal dialogue or hearing another person's voice reading the affirmation." It certainly works for me!

## Make It Personal

The more personal the affirmation, the more effective it is. That's why those positive statements that read more like bumper stickers don't work so well here. Phrases like "Dance Like No One's Watching" or "You Miss 100 Percent of the Shots You Don't Take" are best left to mouse pads and coffee mugs. You must really believe what you're saying. Authenticity and realism are important here. Studies show that completely unobtainable affirmations might have the opposite effect, leaving the affirmer feeling inadequate and, well, less happy than they were beforehand. And remember, if one part of life isn't working out so well, we can draw energy from focusing on other successes.

Focus on your actual qualities and traits or sincere, obtainable goals. Rather than saying, "I am grateful for having the natural physique of a gold medal–winning Olympic gymnast" (unless you really do), you might say, "I'm grateful for my body, for my health, and what it helps me achieve," or even "I love my strong legs and my magnificent elbows, and how I can open a pickle jar in one move."

## *Think Big and Small*

Another trick when making your affirmations is to think about scale. They don't all have to be about winning awards or ringing the bell at the New York Stock Exchange. As much as I want you to think big, I want you to think small, too. Through one of his social media posts, Donald Miller, a supersmart business coach around 750,000 of us follow online, turned me on to the work of Stanford University psychologist Carol Dweck. As a young researcher, Dweck noticed how some children met challenges and failures with ease, while others struggled. "I've always been interested . . . in why some children wilt and shrink back from challenges and give up," she told *The Atlantic* in 2016, "while others avidly seek challenges and become even more invested in the face of obstacles."

She identified what she called a fixed mindset, a belief that our abilities are predetermined and set in stone, and a growth mindset, a belief that our abilities can grow and improve through effort. Spoiler alert: the kids who had the growth mindset were far more likely to succeed. Of course, it's a little more complicated in real life; none of us are 100 percent fixed- or growth-mindset all the time, and gold stars just for effort alone mean sometimes our kids come to see praise as a consolation prize.

But Miller uses Dweck's discoveries in such a clever way. Through his own "self-talk," the dialogue he has with himself—or rather, his affirmations—he is working to stop praising himself for his big accomplishments and begin praising himself for his effort instead. "Great effort in passing on those potato chips," he says, or "great effort in showing up on time to get your writing session done." To him, these small moments of praise add up and give him momentum: the feel-good "dopamine hit" we get from being praised shouldn't just be for those big accomplishments—the small ones need our attention, too. In this way, he says, "You get hooked on making progress," which is something I'm all for!

## How to Avoid Self-Sabotage

I love how affirmations can help protect us, not just from the snark of others, but from our own negative thoughts. They are particularly useful in guarding against self-sabotage. Claude M.

Steele's self-affirmation theory reminds us that, in strengthening our self-belief through affirmation, we are more likely to roll our eyes at negative suggestions than take them to heart. Those bitchy comments you give yourself won't land like they used to.

But self-sabotage is tricky, and developing curiosity here is key. It can take many forms, from procrastination to staying in bed all day, to introducing yourself in negative terms (for example, you're the "hot mess" of your friendship circle)—and especially blaming yourself when something goes wrong. It can be painful to unpick, but a good starting point is to ask yourself, "How am I contributing to my own unhappiness?" Then create an affirmation that pushes a different point of view. It might take a beat, but you'll get there; I know you will.

## How to Raise Your Happiness Baseline

Although creating personalized, meaningful affirmations is essential, there is a happy exception to this rule. Scientist, author, broadcaster, and self-proclaimed "badass" Hannah Fry has a phrase—just five words long—she says can improve your happiness. I was skeptical when I first heard this claim but, girl, she is onto something!

Fry has written about the theory of something called hedonic adaptation, the idea that all of us—no matter how good we feel in one moment, or how bad—will eventually drift back to our original baseline of happiness. This hidden baseline is pretty much set and takes real effort to change, or so the theory goes.

Hedonic adaptation supports the idea that, as our brain imprints our experiences and structures itself accordingly, no matter what joy or pain we experience, we'll probably end up back in the same place. We could just accept this fact, but Fry thinks there's real opportunity here—and so do I.

We must work on raising this baseline, rewiring the brain, and that's just what positive affirmations are all about. So what's the line that Fry says appears to have a "universal positive effect on happiness"? It's a sentence she claims "you should say to yourself as often as you possibly can" as an affirmation; and I can see why. Those magic words of hers? *These are the good days.* It's just perfect, isn't it? Present tense, connecting you with the here and now, and punchy with gratitude. These are the good days.

## The Best Women Talk to Themselves

Of course, I'm not the only woman to talk to herself in times of stress. At the 2024 Paris Olympics, US gymnast Suni Lee dazzled with her floor routine and won a bronze medal for her performance (to go with her gold from the 2020 Tokyo Olympics and countless other awards—oh, and at Paris, she was just twenty-one years old). Like all Olympians, she had had a challenging journey, but perhaps more so because Suni was diagnosed with a kidney condition in 2023. Before her final turn, a routine to "Eye of the Untold Her" by pop violinist Lindsey Stirling, Suni was tied for fourth place. Could she do it?

I remember watching on TV and seeing an emotional Suni moments before she stepped out onto the mat. She was murmuring to herself. The camera caught it, and I immediately thought, *Those are affirmations!* Moments later after an incredible, powerful performance, she won a medal! Soon, the clip was all over TikTok and Instagram, and Suni's affirmations seemed to include "You got this," "This is for me," and "Without a doubt." Go, Suni!

For this chapter, I reached out to another talk-to-herself expert, Lacee Green. Based in California, she's a trainer, coach, mom, and just an all-around major motivating force. She's also a great friend and joy in human form (not an overstatement). We've shared the stage at a few events (we do a bit where Lacee invites me to do a high five, only she's a statuesque goddess and I'm only five-foot-something, so I can never reach!), and I really trust her opinion. I've always wondered how Lacee keeps up her incredible, vivacious energy and was fascinated to discover that affirmations are part of it. I asked her how she uses them in her daily life.

"One thing that has helped me is starting every day with a positive mindset, so I make sure I'm getting in that rhythm each morning," Lacee said. "We're both moms, right? We're both business owners, we're very busy, and things are going to come at you, so you have to prepare."

To do this, Lacee has crafted her own, quirky affirmation trick—it's a simple and effective way to Mind Up and a daily practice that's all her own (and easy to do yourself!), and it's powered by one thing.

"At any point in our lives, we can choose gratitude," she said. "It's not always easy. Especially if something really crappy happens and it's hard to gather up all those 'Oh, find the joy, amen, hallelujah, I'm so happy' feelings. But in most of life's moments, you can choose gratitude, so that's what I focus on.

"The way I do this is, before my feet hit the floor, I touch my thumb to each of my fingers in turn and think or say ten things I'm grateful for. I try to do this without fail. It's funny because sometimes, every once in a while, I'll forget and pull my feet back before they hit the floor really quick. I can't start my day without doing it!"

What are Lacee's things to be grateful for? "Number one always is just 'Praise God that my eyes were open that morning!' That's always the first one, and then it's always my son, my mom, my dad, my family, my health, you know, the big things in all our lives." I love this idea: using affirmations to build a positive mindset by underlining the things you already feel immense gratitude for. The brain loves this kind of thing. "Then, the tenth one is always something silly or ridiculous, like 'I'm grateful for those pink sprinkles on that cupcake,' or 'Praise God for good deodorant.' Just something ridiculous to remind you to not take everything too serious and to always come back to being present."

## MIND UP

I call this—the grateful feeling for those sprinkles or that magical deodorant—the extraordinary ordinary. It's the capacity to see (and take pleasure from) the wonder in the most everyday things in life, and I just love that idea. In our affirmations, we might very well be grateful for those core things: we're grateful to be alive, grateful for the people in our lives, and grateful for who we are, but we sometimes forget to be grateful for the pink sprinkles. Lacee's tenth thing is important because we need to keep our eye on life's little pleasures, or we might just miss them.

Think about whatever it is that brings you a little bit of joy. Maybe you're grateful for a delicious cup of coffee, grateful those flowers bloomed right outside your window, or grateful that it's Taco Tuesday tonight. Remember, those small ideas add up.

So Lacee does her affirmations and is in her positive mindset before her feet hit the floor—but what then? What has her version of Mind Up brought to her daily life?

"The main thing I've learned, and something I talk about with my clients, is that we are not our emotions, and we can try to respond versus react to everything life throws at us." I asked Lacee to go a little deeper: What did she mean by responding rather than reacting to life? Then she really went there: "Andrea, I know neither you nor I expected to be separated and single moms. You didn't see your life playing out that way, nor did I, and yet here we are in the joy of our life! Had those things not happened, I wonder if we would be at this point? But through it all, I learned to respond and not react," she went on.

"And I think that takes time. That's why I really love fitness as a metaphor for life. You don't go from lifting the two-and-a-half-pound dumbbell to the fifty-pound dumbbell overnight. It's a process."

She's right. Neither of us expected to go through our separations and be single moms, but we learned how to respond to our problems, rather than react. We put the time in, with effort and consistency, and we took our power back. And both of us are now on the path we want to be on. "I'm grateful for where I am in my life," said Lacee, "like I'm grateful to be right here in this moment with you right now!" We both laughed—see what I mean about being joy in human form?

## How to Level Up Your Affirmations

Take your affirmations up a notch with these smart, supercharged ideas.

### *It's Okay to Take a Shortcut*

Let's cut to the chase: while affirmations help create an optimistic mindset over time, my shortcut to this mental state is the phrase Mind Up. It reminds me to get back into my gratitude zone and my positive way of thinking. Mind Up is an acknowledgment of the power within me to get shit done.

## MIND UP

Mind Up is also a phrase I use in my parenting. No one wants to hear their mom go on and on with a life lecture (and, truth be told, no mom wants to do it, either), so, in general, I try to lecture less and instead encourage my girls to discover solutions themselves. I want them to find their own answers, to build and maintain their own paths, because I know this will be essential to them long-term. And so, after listening to whatever the problem is, I often remind my girls that they can probably figure this out by themselves: "Mind Up, girl!" which is my way of saying, "I believe in you, and you should, too!"

For my kids, the Mind Up technique is so ingrained that all I need to do is say the words "Mind Up" when I can tell they are feeling down, frustrated, or in a bad mood. They take a deep breath and are already on their way to recovery (girls, if you're reading this, I am so, so proud of you for doing this, even if you often accompany it with an eye roll!).

When I'm exhausted, or if I am in a bad or anxious mood, which is rare, Mind Up resets me. I don't get negative very often and, before Mind Up, I struggled to shake it off because the feeling was so unfamiliar. Mind Up reminds me to stay in the game. I'll tell myself, "Girl, you've got to get your ass up. You've got to move because you've got this vision, this dream of the future; you've got to do it!" Breathwork helps, stretching, too, and movement is essential, but affirmations are what really shifts my mindset.

## Okay, Fine—Write It Down

Recording and listening to your own affirmations in your own voice is key, but you may find other variations that work for you. Here's one I like: Write a simple, positive message on a small slip of paper (remember from chapter 4, there *is* immense power in handwriting). Stick it next to your bed or on your desk or in a small notebook you carry throughout the day—even on your bathroom mirror or on your phone. I have a list of words and phrases that resonate with me, give me a boost, whether I am repeating them to myself during my morning meditations or tagging them above my desk at work:

> I am resilient.
> I stay the course.
> I am so damn worthy.
> I am strong.
> I give it my full-out effort.
> Fight through the fear.
> I keep my chin up.
> Others do not determine my value.
> Others do not determine my choices.
> Others do not determine my happiness.
> I have something unique to offer the world.

In one of the most challenging moments in my life, affirmations and visualizations were all I had. I now know that the habit of speaking, listening, and repeating your affirmations, and closing your eyes and visualizing them coming true, has incredible power.

If you're not taking a few moments every day to think about the things you're grateful for, and where you want to be in life, well, there are better ways of living. Let's turn to one of the greatest thinkers of the modern age, Ferris Bueller—I believe he said it best. At the end of cult teen movie *Ferris Bueller's Day Off* (1986), after the wild adventures of the day, Ferris leaves us with an incredibly wise observation: "I've said it before, and I'll say it again," he says, "life moves pretty fast. You don't stop and look around once in a while, you could miss it." I wholeheartedly agree.

## Taking the Next Step

Often I do not update my affirmations for months, or until a new goal or focus is present, but it's good to refresh them once in a while. Just keep it simple: record it, then replay as many times as you need to throughout the day when you find yourself drifting into a negative headspace. Think of this as a mini meditation session or a quick mental recharge. It's like you just drank a cocktail that brings you back to that place of positive thinking.

Whenever I'm struggling, I play back these recordings—not just once, but multiple times a day, whenever I need hope or reassurance. I put my phone down, sit quietly, press play, listen, and just breathe. I strongly recommend headphones or earbuds, which give an intimacy and depth to your playback. As I listen, I make sure I am active in my thoughts; I visualize my successes, big and small, and I think about what I'm grateful for. As my own voice guides me, I think about my girls, about the love in my life. I think about my healthy body and my healthy mind.

And when my affirmations come to focus on the future, I visualize the things I hope for, like the day I see this book on display in my favorite bookstore (and jump up and down with delight until I'm politely asked to leave!). Perhaps my mind will wander, and that's okay: hearing my own voice will help me refocus.

Back in my crisis zone, the more I used Mind Up, the easier everything became—my breathwork, stretching and movement, my eating, planning, and bedtime rituals—because I had refocused my mind and overridden those self-limiting thoughts in my brain. When your affirmations are personal, punchy, and possible and you really believe them, don't be afraid to put them into action.

## Forget the Sparkles—Wait for the Shine

A brief, final word about waiting it out in the gloom versus the get-up-and-go of positive thinking. Although I always try to avoid negativity, not everything has to be fought with instant optimism, joy, and sparkles. Sometimes, life truly takes an awful turn, and it's okay to feel your feelings. Think of it this way: while a more positive approach isn't going to cure cancer, its relationship to breathwork, stretching, getting into your challenge zone, eating well, good mental health, and a successful sleep practice—all of which have scientifically proven positive effects—should not be underestimated. Optimism is a clear route to achieving your goals, protecting your health, and improving your life—and affirmations are a compelling way to get there.

In my experience, acknowledging your emotions—whatever they are—can only be a good thing. I want my positive thinking to evolve and to grow naturally rather than be forced. Plus, affirmations work best when you really believe them. You might stay in that dark place for a while, and you might need to. But when you're ready, take it from me: affirmations are a truly effective tool to help lift yourself up mentally, and soon you'll start to shine.

Lacee Green told me, "If you always allow yourself to think of the worst-case scenario, would you at least love yourself enough to allow the idea of things turning out better than you could ever imagine? Even if you can't see what that might look like right this second, you have to admit, it's still possible. Know you're not at your final destination. When you can do that, man, that's life-changing." Neither of us spoke for a moment.

That is exactly what I did when I was going through the worst time of my life. It was like everything around me was falling apart, and not just my personal life, but my business, too. In that dark moment I remember thinking—or affirming, rather: *Well, this can't be the end of your story, baby girl! This is not your final chapter or even your middle chapter; it's just one chapter, and you've got so much ahead of you.* It fired up that old confidence I'd had as a child.

Recently, I asked my mom about this childhood confidence and where it came from, and her answer was very Maybelline. "You were born with it." She laughed. "You've been like this since you were a baby!" This feels true to me. Before my relationship breakdown, I had always been very confident in who I was, what I could do, and my value. I found my purpose very early on in life; I was good at dancing, I had a natural ability for it, and I was able to combine it with hard work and consistent effort over time. I worked my ass off and it got me places. But then, I lost myself for a while.

As I pieced my life back together, recording and replaying my affirmations seemed to draw out that same strong, energized, and optimistic Midwestern girl. I had finally found my way back to her.

When in doubt, Mind Up.

## daily practice #7

# breathe it out

*letting go of the scaries,
and setting yourself up
for a skillful sleep*

> **WHAT WILL I BE DOING?**
> Physical and mental preparation
> so you can sleep with skill.
>
> **HOW LONG WILL IT TAKE?**
> 2 minutes, minimum.
>
> **WHEN DO I DO IT?**
> Right at the end of the day.
>
> **AND WHAT WILL I ACHIEVE?**
> No-fail sleep skills to prep your body and mind for the best sleep of your life. With a little consistency, you could be the most accomplished sleeper ever!

How skilled are you at sleeping?

Wait, you thought it was about just lying there and doing nothing? Nope! It's an active process that takes preparation, consistency, and—yes—skill. And so, Daily Practice #7, our final activity of the day, is about learning how to set yourself up to sleep with skill, aka getting the most benefit from those nighttime hours.

Now, I know some of you might have raw talent in this area. You'll no doubt be thinking, *Oh, honey, if there were an Olympics for sleeping, I'd be up on that podium.* But most of us—in fact, many of the women I work with—have a complicated relationship with sleep. So I want you to rethink your approach to bedtime, stop winging your snooze sessions, create an end-of-day ritual you'll be able to do with your eyes closed, and banish the Midnight Scaries for good.

For Daily Practice #7, we'll be reframing sleep as a skill to master and preparing for bedtime—training for it, even—as an essential task that must be done with care and patience. Failing consistently here can have terrible health implications . . . but succeeding? Well, it improves just about everything.

I get it: you should be able to sleep well, naturally, no effort needed. And that would be true if our minds weren't so busy, and our bodies and brains weren't so overstimulated. This is why you shouldn't just assume that when you turn off the lights you will just fall asleep.

In learning to sleep skillfully, you'll be preparing your environment, switching off stimuli, and using breathwork (now that you're doing this every morning, you will be a pro at night) to mentally declutter so you can sleep more soundly.

## Why Sleep Is So Important

If you know me, you know not to mess with my sleep! I'm very protective of it. I travel lots and can get by on very few hours (and still have a great day when I wake up), but I really cherish my sleep, and I've learned the hard way that my bedtime is the foundation of my overall health, happiness, and well-being. If I don't get the sleep I need in terms of hours and quality, I'm not my best self.

And it's not just me. Research has shown that women have more difficulty going to sleep and staying asleep than men. For that, we can thank a number of things. First up, hormones: sleep problems are more likely in the days leading up to your period, or if you're perimenopausal or menopausal (cue hot flashes and night sweats), and sleep can also be tough in the third trimester for pregnant women. Conditions like fibromyalgia and chronic pain conditions—again, more common in women—are associated with sleep loss, too. Even societal expectations on us as perfect professionals, mothers, partners, caregivers, and domestic goddesses can weigh in here, with our schedules invading our sleep time. If we're not careful, it really adds up. Cumulatively, chronic sleep loss and sleep disorders can mean an increased risk of hypertension, diabetes, obesity, depression, heart attack, and stroke. So what's a girl to do to get a little shut-eye?

Healthy sleep at a healthy time is critical—we know this because we can see what happens when we don't get it. We're a mess. Deep sleep is the body's repair mode: your hormones regulate, your immune system refreshes, your heart experiences less strain, and your brain rewires itself. For some, lack of sleep is the missing ingredient to their strength-building or weight-loss journey, the reason why they're just not progressing. And for kids and teens, sleep is essential for growth and brain development.

Although you can't "make up" missed sleep (of course, if you're tired during the day, there's a nap for that), there is a way to counteract the occasional bad night—and as we've already done it for an earlier Daily Practice, you'll soon be a pro! A team of researchers in China analyzed health data from 92,000 participants in the United Kingdom; just over half were female aged between forty and seventy-three, and each wore a techy wristband tracking their sleep and physical activity over one week. The study took many years to complete, but the results published in 2023 suggest that you can wipe out the long-term effects of missing sleep with exercise. Sleeping poorly is often associated with higher mortality, and the Chinese researchers were looking for ways in which exercise might shield us from bad health outcomes. They found people who exercised lots did not have an increased risk, *even when they slept less than six hours*. Rough night? Daily Practice #3, Just Press Play, will help heal the damage.

Still, we can't have an excellent workout if we haven't slept well—we need to do both successfully. Sleeping badly compromises our health, but just *knowing* how important it is doesn't ensure a good night's sleep. I know it can be frustrating when you have the best of intentions but your body won't play along. What if I go to bed and don't feel tired?

The necessary ingredients for restful sleep are keeping to your schedule, avoiding stimulation (from screens to caffeine), being active during the day, and creating the right physical and mental conditions to cue your brain and body to power down and Breathe It Out.

## How to Do It

Although Daily Practice #7 has breathwork at its core, your sleep setup—preparing your mind, body, and environment—is essential.

### Switching Off

First, let's get ready for bed by preparing our brain and body for a restful night. After a big day, many of us head over to Netflix or fire up Instagram (pick your poison) to relax. And sometimes we lose track of time. It's natural to want to slow down when we can, and I'm all for it. But I know I'm not the only person to look up and realize it's late, season two is already auto playing, or that the infinite scroll proved alarmingly close to infinite. *I'd better get to bed now*, you think, *or I'm in trouble*. You head upstairs, brush your teeth . . . and somehow keep scrolling with your free hand. You get into bed and turn off the light before a final few minutes of scrolling—just a couple more emotional dog rescue clips and neck pillow ads.

Oh, and once that phone is finally put to bed, your brain stays switched on. Now it's playing all of your favorite worries over and over in your head, and you find it nearly impossible to turn it off.

This is, I am sad to say, terrible for your sleep cycle. You're overstimulating your brain, and when you finally make it under the covers, you've set yourself up for some very shoddy shut-eye (try saying that when you're tired). And worse, it sets you up to experience the same knock-down, drag-out day tomorrow, followed by the same attempt to chill.

The aim here is to adopt a practice of progressive relaxation to cue your brain that sleep is on its way. So, everything you do here for Daily Practice #7 will be about slowing down, calming your body and mind, and following your own tailored-to-you routine to bring you sleep success.

In a way, your night routine can be thought of as prep for your morning routine: Want to feel refreshed and ready to kick ass tomorrow? Set the tone *tonight*. But, if I can impart only one lesson in this book, it's this: Do The Thing. Consistency is everything for locking in healthy habits—and treating sleep seriously.

## Breathing Out

Back when it all hit the fan, I used my breath for emergency relief. In the first chapter, I describe how I was able to harness breath-power in a real moment of need. At the time, I had no idea the years I'd spent actively using breath in both my dance training and Pilates career would come in so handy, and while a little unexpected breathwork got me out of a tough spot, there are more ways to use this essential skill. What we started with Daily Practice #1, our first ritual of the day, we can now repeat with Daily Practice #7, but in a completely different way.

Breath is your built-in power tool, and just as we can charge it up and use it to strengthen, draw in positivity, and encourage an energetic focus to start the day, we can also use it to wind down and really let go of things, emotionally and physically, before we turn out the lights.

Just as the day began with fixing your intention and drawing in your breath, you will now let go of the day behind you and breathe out gently, releasing negative thoughts. (Remember how easy breathwork is? You're already doing it!).

I take a moment to focus, and as I inhale, I'll really acknowledge my worries, something like: "Oh my God, I don't know what I'm doing with my life. I want to move to New York. But I don't know if that's good for the kids . . ." And then, as I slowly exhale, I let go of the emotional stress and remind myself I'll figure it all out in time.

I acknowledge my worries on the inhale and "release them" on the exhale.

What I mean by "release them" is that I just let those thoughts dissipate; I let them drift into nothingness along with my exhale.

Your bedtime exercise takes two minutes, and it's called Breathe It Out. After tucking your bookmark back in your book, finishing your chamomile tea, and stifling those yawns, you are ready for the last step in your bedtime ritual: relaxing breathwork.

## breathe it out

**WHAT IT DOES**
Quiets the mind

**TIME IT TAKES**
2 minutes (or more if you're feeling it)

**HOW TO DO IT**
Just as the day began with fixing your intention and drawing in your breath, you will let go of the day behind you and breathe out gently. For a count of 4, breathe in what is still holding your attention from the day, focusing on a particular worry, frustration, or concern—whatever's putting a bee in your bonnet—and then exhale slowly to a count of 8, releasing it, and giving yourself a little grace as you do it. Visualize the problem disappearing—you can't solve it now. Let it go.

## Deal with the Sunday Scaries

What's important to remember, and a little counterintuitive, I admit, is that exhaling isn't a solution to these worries. I wish it was!

There is no higher consciousness third eye opening going on here, nor do I exhale and think, *Done! I'm over that and I will never think about it again!* I just accept that my worrisome thing is going to be something I need to work on, and I remind myself there's nothing I can do about it at that moment. Am I going to get up right that second, fly to New York, and see how I feel? No, that would be ridiculous. No one is going to solve all their problems just before bed. I work on accepting that.

Then, for my next round of breathwork, I might move on to another thing that's on my mind. *How did I handle that situation with my daughter?* I might think. *How can I do better?*

Again, I allow myself some grace. If your worry is something similar, acknowledge it and remind yourself that tomorrow maybe you'll try something different. But right now? That's enough. No more guilt, no more thinking about it. So, you got this one wrong; it doesn't mean you're an awful person! But if you ignore it, shut it out, and leave it unexamined, it's still there. And let me tell you, for many of us, it shows up again later. It shows up in my sleep, it shows up in my stress, and it shows up the next morning when I wake. Just when I'm about to start breathwork, stretching, and my movement session and I want to be the most powerful in my mindset, I'll find I'm in a funk because of all the worries I shoved away hours earlier.

A middle-of-the-night hack I've used in the past—when I haven't quite achieved my Breathe It Out routine and I'm suddenly awake in the moonlight, stressed—is that I'll get up and write down what's bothering me, adding whatever it is to tomorrow's Daily Practice #4 Do The Thing list. By doing that, I'm letting my brain know that I'll get to it later, it will be taken care of, and I can go back to the job of sleeping well. It really helps.

## Putting Your Worries to Bed

So you've prepared your body and your environment for sleep, but what about sleeping skillfully? What about mentally decluttering your mind?

For me, I'm a big nighttime thinker. I can lie there wondering about everything and anything, things I want to achieve, places I want to visit, but if I'm not careful, the heavy stuff can creep in, too. Thinking all those worrisome thoughts so late in the day is like having the Sunday Scaries, only every day of the week.

Insomnia, the catchall term for sleep trouble (problems falling or staying asleep, or if your sleep is low quality), is more common than it should be. My Tools of the Trade checklist (which we'll get to later in this chapter) addresses your body's physical needs, but we also need to prep our emotional ones, too. What will fix that churn of thoughts, memories, and fears?

Last time I couldn't sleep I woke up at 1:45 AM, and for two whole hours my mind went wherever it wanted to. *Should I move back to New York? What would happen to the kids? Wait, what was that noise? Was that a gunshot? Nope, I'm being silly . . . But should I move them to a city where there are gunshots?* And then, later, it got existential. *Why are we here?* And finally: *Why did I say that embarrassing thing last week?* and *Did I forget to buy matcha?* I really went there.

I was ruminating. Women tend to ruminate, often unproductively, more than men, and you're even more likely to do it if you have a perfectionist outlook. That's why I think allowing for a little self-love at the end of the day is essential. I'd had some of these negative thoughts before bed, but I'd immediately shut them down, thinking that was the right thing to do. I soon realized that by not dealing with my night thoughts, by not even acknowledging them, I was setting myself up to fail. They would come anyway, crawling through my dreams like zombies. Or worse, Deb would appear. That's the name I gave to my inner critical voice. In fact, it's probably time you met her.

## *Not Now, Deb*

A few years ago, while on vacation in Scottsdale, my partner booked us both a round of golf. Although I played a little when I was younger, I was only then getting back into the sport and finding my groove. It's a slow, thoughtful game, played in gorgeous surroundings, and I remember us laughing all day in the sunshine: I was loving every moment. For those who don't know their putter from their wedge, on some golf courses, when you're in a twosome, you get paired with another twosome. Now, it could be a match made in heaven or pretty much the opposite, so you either have a great game or it's like pulling teeth. On this day, my partner and I were paired up with a husband and his wife; let's call her Deb. And Deb was not happy to be paired with us, not one little bit. She harrumphed her way around the course, sighing and tutting every time I swung for the ball. She seemed almost angry to be out on the green with such an amateur.

Now, I'm still working on my handicap, and I am gradually getting better, but as much as I take the sport seriously, we also like to have fun when we golf. I was determined to break the ice with Deb, but she was a hard nut to crack. We remembered we had a little music speaker with us and, with me nodding my encouragement, my partner asked, "Hey, Deb, what's your favorite song?" She turned toward him, rolling her eyes, and simply said, "I don't like music." I was shocked. That's like saying you don't like trees! Or you don't like to breathe! "What do you mean you don't like music?" he asked playfully, a big, friendly grin on his face. "Come on, you gotta like one song!" But Deb was having none of it, not from us, anyway. She shook her head. "I don't like music, I don't listen to music, and that's that." Then she picked up her putter and putted right off.

My partner and I laughed about it over lunch and joked that we don't want to be a "Deb" about things. Maybe Deb was just having a bad day and, of course, she has her own story, but she—or rather, her attitude—really stuck in my mind. After our awkward afternoon together, I thought about Deb for days, and slowly the idea of her became connected to my own negative emotions, giving them character and taking on her name. If I'm feeling anxious or lacking motivation, I think, *Oh no, Deb is here*. Or if I'm feeling a little cranky and tired: you guessed it, it's Deb. In fact, don't we all have a little Deb inside us, telling us "I don't want to do that" or "I don't like music"? Deb became my own critical inner voice.

For me, giving that voice a name really helped. When I hear myself saying, "No, you can't," or "Do not wear that; you look absolutely ridiculous," or "Are you kidding me? You're not capable of that; that's for other people, not for someone like you," I immediately say, "Oh, wait a second there, Deb, not today." That little Deb voice always pops up when things are tough, from a busy day with work and family pressures, to an intense movement class, even a steep weekend hike. "Not now, Deb," I'll say. "Not now."

Back in my bedroom, in the early hours of the morning, Deb was in full force, but I decided that, if I was ever going to sleep, I had to finally entertain her, just a little. And it worked. "Girl, if you shut down those thoughts, you can't just expect them to go away," I told myself. "They'll haunt you. But if you address those worries before you go to bed, then they've had their attention. They've done their little dance for you. And they won't wake you in the night." Finally, I had found my solution. To get rid of my night thoughts, I had to listen to them—and it really works.

To recap: Daily Practice #7 is about rethinking how you sleep, switching off stimuli, preparing your environment, and using breathwork to help acknowledge—and let go of—any worries or concerns. Nail these three elements and you've completed daily Practice #7 with style!

## Level Up Your Sleep Schedule

Here's how you can go even further and put everything you've just learned together into a life-changing nightly routine.

Here's mine.

### *1. Set Your Phone to "Do Not Disturb"*

We all know the stress response triggered when we hear that digital *ding*! At least an hour before bed, switch your phone to "Do Not Disturb," or customize it so the setting turns itself on at the same time every workday evening. I do this, and it's a game changer.

### *2. Turn Off Your Computer and Your TV*

If you do have to work online after the sun has gone down, use blue light filtering glasses (there are some fabulous and inexpensive ones out there) or a nighttime screen setting. Blue light—the wavelength that glows from our phones, tablets, laptop screens, and even energy-efficient lighting—boosts attention and even mood. Blue light is everywhere, even in sunlight, but what makes us more alert during the day can be pretty disruptive at night, and it's our screens that are the culprits. The key here is melatonin, the hormone essential for the normal running of our circadian rhythm (our body's daily biological schedule). Simply put, melatonin is suppressed when exposed to that blue wavelength.

What's more, watching anything—especially anything highly stimulating—will wake up your brain just when you need it to be as calm as possible. The finale of your favorite prestige-TV drama, with all its twists and turns, might just have to be scheduled a little earlier next time.

## 3. Eat Dinner at Least Three Hours Before Bed

I know that's early for some and might seem like the craziest idea ever if you're from a country where eating as late as possible is a cultural institution. (This is a good time to mention that my amazing dad is French, and he'll be rolling his eyes at this advice!) But that's how long your food will take to digest. Any pre-bed snack will make it harder to fall asleep and stay asleep. If you are very hungry and hunger pangs will otherwise keep you awake, eat only a small amount of protein and an even smaller amount of complex carbs together (such as a small portion of unsweetened Greek yogurt and half an apple or banana), as this could reduce the chance of an insulin spike.

## 4. Take a Warm Shower (or a Bath if You Have the Time)

It's a traditional sleep remedy for a reason: doing so will actually lower your core temperature, which is a signal for your circadian rhythm that bedtime is coming. Science backs this up: it was Shahab Haghayegh, now an instructor at Harvard Medical School, who tested the idea that a warm soak in the tub an hour or two before bed (with or without bubbles—the study's unclear on that part) can bring on sleep success.

Back when he was a student at the University of Texas at Austin, Haghayegh was going to bed after midnight, waking for class at 8 AM, yet soon found himself completely sleep starved and feeling awful. Making time for a soothing nighttime soak in the tub really helped, so Haghayegh and other researchers conducted an analysis of sleep studies to see if they could find out why—and their discovery really made a splash. They published their results in 2019, identifying a link between warm baths and showers and better, more successful sleep, even suggesting a little tub time could replace sleeping meds for some people.

Your body temperature needs to lower slightly to be able to snooze well. It naturally cools before bedtime, with heat moving out from your core and toward your hands and feet, where it burns off. A warm bath or shower helps push this process along—you might feel all cozy and warm after a bath, but your inner temperature is actually dropping. You've done it: you successfully tricked your body into getting into the sleep zone!

Epsom[1] salts are a good addition to your bath even if the science around its benefits is a little patchy. Rich in magnesium, a natural sleep aid, and a soother of aching muscles, Epsom salts feel great, though the jury is out on how well we absorb minerals transdermally, or through our skin. But enough of us in the fitness world love Epsom salt baths to strongly suggest a benefit, and its role as a post-workout recovery practice is pretty solid in the fitness community. Remember to shower off afterward (the salts can irritate sensitive skin), and then enjoy the deliciously sleepy feeling that follows.

Light a candle, use a fragrant bath oil (more on that later), play your favorite calming music: ultimately, a bath or shower before bed—even a quick one—is an opportunity to relax, be mindful, and treat yourself. To me, having a bath most nights feels like a luxury, and who doesn't want that?

## 5. Have a Cup of Unsweetened Herbal Tea

I especially like chamomile, valerian, or lemon balm tea. I know you know this, but no matter how good a post-dinner espresso may sound, no caffeine! You should also avoid alcohol within four hours of bedtime, so no espresso martini, either. According to Dr. Jennifer Martin, a psychologist and professor of medicine at the University of California, Los Angeles, alcohol is "initially sedating, but as it's metabolized, it's very activating," joining the list of those things you think will calm you but actually does the opposite.

## 6. Read a Book Before Sleep

(Maybe this one?) Ideally, read in a comfortable bedroom chair—wait to get in bed until you are really ready to sleep. This helps your body know that, once lying down, it's safe to switch off.

## 7. Try a Bedtime Meditation

From chapter 2, you will know that meditation has mind-calming powers. We've already discussed the relationship between morning stretching and meditation, but taking a moment to meditate before bed—either sitting quietly or lying down—can help you release any intrusive thoughts and feelings of the day.

## 8. Lights Out

A dark, cool room is important for getting quality sleep—see my Tools of the Trade checklist for more. Sweet dreams!

## Sleep Like a Kid After a Day at the Beach

I'm very mindful in how I set up my own nighttime habits, and being a mom, I know how important routine is for my children to have a restful sleep. I draw on that direct experience as a parent, through lots of trial and tantrums, in creating my perfect end-of-day ritual.

If you're a parent—or if you've ever just been a kid—this will resonate.

With our younger kids we don't just say, "See ya, peace out, good night!" We make efforts to create a routine, knowing this will pay off in the long run: bath time, putting on PJs, low lighting, and story time. Done consistently, it means our kids know just what to expect, and their bodies and minds are all set to shut down for the night.

With my girls, our nighttime routine has been simple: they get a heads-up a half hour before getting ready for bed. Then it's time for them to wash up (now that they are older, it's all about skin care time), brush their teeth and hair, and get into their cozies. Then I come up and give them a squeeze—it's wonderfully intimate and loving—and it's lights out. The only rule is that there should be no devices in their room at night.

Not only am I training them for great sleep (I really, really want them to master this skill), but after the girls go to bed, I have a bonus hour or so of "me time" before I go to sleep, too. Having a consistent routine night after night not only makes babies and children feel comforted and nurtured—it works for parents, too. Of course, our routine wasn't always quite this locked down. As a mom, I have more than a few "bedtime stories," but we got there in the end!

We go to great efforts to ritualize sleep for kids, with each step carefully planned and carried out to prepare them for the night ahead (that old cliché of parents doing literally anything to get their kids to sleep is true!), but we don't do that for ourselves as adults. Why not? Instead, we're on the phone, sipping from a glass of wine, clicking through endless streamer menus, and then we turn off the TV and slump into bed minutes later, hoping for the best (and probably forgetting our retainer).

## Bedtime Means Business

Another perspective: when you have an important meeting, you don't walk in unprepared. You organize your notes, you know what you hope to achieve, and you have a plan for how you are going to achieve it. You don't come running in five minutes before the meeting is going to start and think you can wing it (well, maybe this has happened once or twice, but it's never the best-case scenario). But that's what happens with sleep if you don't have a plan. Learn to use a business mindset: focus on what you want to achieve, use the hours leading up to bedtime to prepare, and set out to nail it.

Preparing your environment for sleep is essential—whether it's an airline seat, a hotel, or your own bed. Even if you are on a budget and can't afford to try them all, it is worth it to think about a small upgrade or two. For example, if you hate your pillow, save up for a really good one. (I did this and invested in a pillow I love. It was worth every penny, as my sleep improved literally overnight.) Overall, bedtime should make you feel good, so invest if you can.

## So You Think You Can Sleep?

No one I know has a busier schedule than Lacey Schwimmer. She's the award-winning professional dancer who quickstepped her way onto *So You Think You Can Dance?* and *Dancing with the Stars* (her paso doble with Lance Bass from NSYNC is the stuff of legends!). She is always working it, always traveling all over the country, always showing up and performing full-out. I'm in awe of her and, over the many years we've been friends, I'd always wondered but never asked: *How the heck does she do it?*

I reached out to Lacey and asked her to come clean about her sleep routine. I wanted to discover what part, if any, sleep plays in her overall approach to healthy, happy living.

"I was around nineteen years old when I started working in television, and back then, sleep was not a priority," she told me. "You just don't want to miss anything! I can't tell you how many nights on *So You Think You Can Dance?* where I maybe had just an hour of sleep and then on TV at 4 AM. But it got really interesting for me, sleep wise, when I was on *Dancing with the*

*Stars.*" On *DWTS*, Lacey was paired with celebrities who often had very little experience dancing. "The stress was far greater because it wasn't me that was being judged: I was in charge of someone else's success."

I know a little of this feeling from my own teaching and coaching; being responsible for someone winning or losing a big TV show would surely pile on the pressure.

"Now, as I'm getting older, and my job is very physical, I have to be rested and show up performance ready. Whether it's performing at Carnegie Hall or in an arena somewhere, or just showing up at a studio to teach children, it's still the same amount of preparation and care that goes into it. When I was younger, I used to think we can always sleep later, right? But now, to be completely performance ready, sleep is essential."

A long career at the very top level of dance has meant that Lacey has learned a thing or two about skillful sleeping—she's had to. "It's about routine, right?" she said. "Creating bedtime rituals that just make you feel centered, calm, and okay with your day. You're not thinking about the next thing; you're just in your own moment, appreciating the time you have, and relaxing."

For Lacey, it all starts with a nighttime bath. "I add relaxing, essential oils. I love lavender; eucalyptus to breathe clearly. Tea tree is good if it's been a nasty day and I need to detox. I also add super high-quality magnesium salts. I always try to make it smell like a spa. You know, where they play that really weird music that you can't ever understand what it is, but you like it."

Can't you just breathe in that aroma right now? And hear that—what is it—whalesong? I'm scheduling some tub time tonight, and you should, too.

Although she might add a little screen time to her end-of-day ritual, Lacey makes a point of picking something that's not too stimulating or something she's seen before, "like *The Office*," said Lacey. "That's what I'm rewatching now. It's like my seventeenth time, but I love it. I love relaxing to podcasts and audiobooks, too.

"I know a lot of people read to unwind, which is fantastic, but I'd struggle," said Lacey. "Since I was about ten years old, I've had ADHD and severe anxiety, and reading doesn't calm me." I agree wholeheartedly that we all need to identify what calms us, and not expect it to look the same across the board.

"I think it's good to know what you like and not force it," I said, and reading is optional! "If it feels like a nonnegotiable, and isn't something that calms you," I went on, "then it has the opposite effect."

Lacey even prioritizes sleep when she's on tour. "Traveling, that's the worst, right? You're not in your own bed. You're in a different time zone, and there's so many stimulating things throughout your day. So, I bring a sleep care package with me: I have my 3D eye mask so my eyelashes don't get smudged, and they have Bluetooth speakers in them so I can block outside noise. I have earplugs, too, and they really work.

"I get my most natural sleep on an airplane. I know that sounds so crazy." It really didn't, I told her, because I sleep well on a plane, too. "I put my noise-canceling headphones on, then my eye mask, and then I have a foot hammock. You know about my foot hammock, right?"

I sure did. Lacey had posted about her favorite in-flight gadgets on Instagram weeks earlier, and she looked like she was at a spa! I bought them all, there and then. But it makes sense to me that Lacey sleeps so well in transit because her approach, which includes preparation (her gadgets) and a focused mindset, creates the perfect conditions for successful sleep—even in such a distracting and stimulating environment.

"I think it's about having balance. And I'm still learning that balance, obviously, but I schedule my time a little differently now. For example, if I'm not working, I like to shut off around 6 PM every night like a grandma!"

So many of us let a bad night's sleep turn us into a crab fest the next day. You're not always going to get those perfect eight or nine hours of sleep, but Daily Practice #7 will put you in the best position possible. Lacey's approach inspires me: prioritizing sleep as much as possible, ritualizing certain aspects, creating a "sleep care package" for when she's on the move, and some happy flexibility and a strong Mind Up attitude when sleep is scarce. Plus, a "grandma night" that involves an aromatic bath and my favorite audiobook? I'm in!

You're almost ready to drop off, I know, but let's finish up with a few final items to consider. Each one is designed to help send you straight to sleep.

## Tools of the Trade

When you're tired, *any* bed seems like it'll do the job—but if you really want quality sleep, there are a few things I recommend (and a few must-haves) to go from just recharging your batteries to waking up feeling truly refreshed.

### *A Supportive Bed*

It is easy to forget how important the bed itself is. If your bed isn't right—if it's too soft or hard—you'll be tossing and turning all night (and visiting a chiropractor all day). It's a personalized purchase, so I recommend trying out your mattress before you buy. You're likely to end up with something medium firm—most people do—so start there.

### *Inviting Linens and Soothing Colors*

Natural fibers like cotton, linen, bamboo, and silk help your skin breathe at night. My bedroom's color palette is all neutral—beige, white, and taupe—for a calm mindset. I recently found my daughter the most deliciously soft bedding (HomeGoods for the win!), which helped her fall asleep much faster.

## A Weighted Blanket

If you have anxiety, this may be for you! Weighted blankets—quilts studded inside with a grid of weights—have become popular in recent years and are based on a therapeutic technique of deep-pressure stimulation. It's like being swaddled.

## The Best Pillow Ever (for You)

Choose pillows that make you feel good when you lie down—everyone has different preferences. A pregnancy pillow can also be helpful for those with chronic backaches or other muscle issues. This one sleep essential offers almost too many options, but with a little research, you'll find the right one for you, whether you're a side, back, or stomach sleeper. Shredded foam seems to keep its volume longer than other filling options, but maybe you're a feather down kind of girl?

## Sleepwear You Absolutely Love

Make sure it's roomy enough for you to move around in as you sleep. Natural fibers are the best for your jammies, and there's absolutely nothing—nothing!—in this world as pleasurable as putting on a pair of crisp cotton PJs for the first time. I will be taking no questions at this time.

## An Aromatherapy Diffuser or Spray

Lavender, ylang ylang, chamomile, sandalwood, bergamot, vetiver, cedarwood, and ginger are among the most popular scents used for sleep. You can also get lavender sprays for your bedding that make your bed smell heavenly, or search for an organic pillow spray that will do the same. Or you can add a few drops of any aromatherapy oil to your bath. I am currently obsessed with my magnesium spray and give a quick mist on my pillow and use on the bottom of my feet every night. Try it, trust me.

## Blackout Curtains

I highly recommend you invest in blackout curtains or, at the very least, a comfortable eye mask. Too much light stimulates cortisol—the stress hormone!—while darkness stimulates your body to produce melatonin. Dr. Phyllis Zee and a team at Northwestern University tested out the relationship between sleep quality and light levels in 2022. They ran a small study with twenty volunteers, tucking them up in bed in a dark room on one night and in a "moderately well-lit" room another night—they wanted to see what would happen just one night without total darkness. After sleeping in the light room, participants had trouble processing sugar the following day compared to their night in the dark, even if they reportedly slept well both nights!

## Climate Control

Even a fan will help. Your bedroom should ideally be somewhere around a cool 65 degrees Fahrenheit. I know, I know, that's a little chilly, but remember how your body cools down to sleep effectively? Give it a go.

## A White Noise Machine

If you live in a big city or need ambient noise, there are great solutions for you—and many of them are free. You can invest in a white noise machine or just look for an ambient noise playlist on your iPhone or a Relaxing White Noise podcast episode (they're eight hours long!). Don't want it playing all night? Set a timer with the "Stop Playing" silent alarm tone.

## A Humidifier

If you live somewhere cold and dry, in my opinion, this is a must. At the time of this writing, quiet, WiFi-controlled "smart" humidifiers are your best bet. For health reasons, remember to rinse and dry it regularly, plus give your humidifier a proper cleaning once or twice a week. Humidifiers hold water at room temperature for days; if you wouldn't drink it from a glass, don't use it in your machine.

Just as we took a deep, energizing inhale at the beginning of the day, we'll exhale here, at bedtime, having prepared our environment, body, and mind for the best sleep ever.

Okay, let's lie down, get comfortable and cozy, and Breathe It Out.

# conclusion
## we're on the trail together

CONCLUSION

While writing this book, I took a weekend trip to Aspen where my friend Lacey (yes, *another* Lacey—I know many and I love them all) invited me on what turned out to be a stunningly beautiful but pretty aggressive mountain hike. It was late spring but felt more like summer, and we were soon sweating as we scrambled over boulders and hoisted ourselves up rocky ledges.

It's part of my job to stay as fit as I can, but moving along a trail at such a steep incline is like being on a runaway StairMaster cranked up to its highest setting. It was unbelievably tough. Plus, we were at high altitude, and at some points, I had to stop every ten seconds or so to catch my breath. That's when Deb started making herself known.

Remember her? The name I gave my own negative thoughts? I could feel her starting to creep in, and I began to doubt if I could really Do The Thing after all. "You should call it a day," Deb said, assuredly, inside my head. "You're not cut out for this."

Now, because Lacey is so experienced, and also just a really great person, I knew I was with someone who could not only help me pace myself, but encourage me, too. I was right: "You can do it," said Lacey, sensing that I was struggling. "Just one baby step at a time, and if you have to stop for ten seconds and catch your breath, stop for ten seconds and catch your breath!" In just a few words, Lacey made it clear she had absolute faith in me. *I don't want to let her down!* I thought, *and I don't want to let myself down!* Those resolutions shut off Deb's voice for good.

## CONCLUSION

I was (and always am) wowed by Lacey; she has done that hike solo many times, without the kind of encouragement she was giving me, and had never given up. I was reminded that it takes an incredible amount of resilience to do something like that on your own. Powered by Lacey's encouragement, her evident personal strength, and my inner badass, it was time to level up and get tough with myself: *You're going to keep going up that trail and all the way to that damn summit.* And I did.

Sometimes, we all need a friend on the trail (especially during those days and weeks that feel like you're on a runaway StairMaster). I realized on the summit of that mountain in Aspen, with the sun on my face and my buddy by my side, that's exactly what I hope *Small Moves, Big Life* might be to you.

Because we're doing this together.

You may be reading this—right at the end of this book—thinking, *I know this!* Or you feel reminded of something you already learned in the past. I would feel very happy if that's what you took from this book. Connecting you with that inner knowledge, that common sense, is really my aim here. If these practices resonate with you because they tap into something you already know—or used to know—then that's wonderful! I hope I've reminded you that these practices are integral to maintain in your daily life to stay at your best and be truly present as you move through the world. I know this because I've lived through it.

Behind these integral practices is a set of essential truths. And what I love most about these ideas—and how they manifest in breathwork, stretching, and preparing your body and mind for sleep, and so on—is their simplicity. They seem familiar because, in some shape or form, they're already part of our lives.

But what I've come to learn, sometimes the hard way, is that the immense, transformative superpowers of these ideas are only unlocked through consistency and effort over time.

Try each one: practice a stretch routine, sit down for breakfast, and breathe out your negative thoughts before bedtime. That alone is great. But the effects of doing them every single day, with full-out effort, will accumulate over time—small moves make a big life, and the results will blow your mind. Great ideas are only great if you really live them, each and every day.

That's why I've made these intentional habits into Daily Practices, that's why each one is just a few minutes long, and that's why I do them myself. They are designed to be lived—every single day—consistently and with authenticity.

At first, you'll wonder if it's working. Life might have felt so stuck and stressful, and the rut you've been in so very deep, that you might need to step out of the ordinary and the everyday to really feel it.

You'll be heading off on a trip, maybe, and instead of the usual anxious anticipation of delays, missed connections, and "Damn, did I forget the handwipes?" you'll notice the sun streaming in through the airport windows. Somehow, in that moment, you'll just feel . . . calm.

CONCLUSION

You'll have a week or two of mini workouts behind you, and you just shifted eight bags of groceries from your car to the kitchen without getting out of breath. In that moment, you realize your strength and stamina have increased. Even your clothes fit differently. You're more flexible and less injury-prone, and you can feel your muscles are just a little more toned. Oh, and something's going on with your skin: it's looking fresh!

Things that might usually irritate you, needling away until you snap—well, they haven't troubled you at all. You find yourself breathing through it; mindful breath is your new go-to when dealing with stress. You're eating a little better, and you're sleeping well, too. You'll laugh at something out loud, and you'll think, *Wow, I haven't done that in a while.* You've identified something in the future you'd like to work toward. Things feel . . . good.

Nothing *huge* has happened (not yet, anyway). No one transforms overnight. But you have a different perspective, and you feel things in a new rhythm. You're on a new path and—I promise you—girl, it will feel great!

When I discovered that breathwork could truly save me in times of stress, that recording affirmations could help rewire my brain for the better, that sitting down for just ten minutes helped me foster a healthier relationship with food, and that there are big benefits to learning to sleep with skill, they were incredible realizations. I tried and tested each one, did them daily, and soon felt their potential; they were like beautiful, powerful little trinkets I put carefully into my jewelry box.

Those trinkets became this book of 7 Daily Practices, and I hope they can help both you and me stay on the trail.

My 7 Daily Practices remain the bedrock of my day. I'm still facing my own challenges, trying to overcome setbacks, and I'm always looking for ways to grow: the trail is ongoing! My own successes in my personal and professional life are pretty much *because* I've consistently performed my 7 Daily Practices, each and every day, seven days a week, for years. In fact, I don't think I could be a single mom and run a business full-time and *not* do them, and I clearly would not have truly survived my divorce and turned my life's trajectory around without learning and exploring these powerful rituals.

Now, a little more real talk: you have a choice.

You don't have to walk the trail. You can choose not to do the 7 Daily Practices. You can stay in that rut, telling yourself every day that, even though you want to set a new course, you need just one more day to put your affairs in order. Nope! This procrastinating has got to stop. No matter how hard it seems, you can break the pattern, but it really must be today, not tomorrow. And it all starts with just two minutes of breathwork—there's nothing easier!

We've already discussed how many of us feel bad spending time on self-care and renewal. We battle feelings of inadequacy, low productivity, and guilt, and our own needs fall by

## CONCLUSION

the wayside. But these 7 Daily Practices—they take just thirty minutes combined—have a pleasing side effect. Do them with full-out effort and you will have more time and energy for yourself and for your loved ones. Just as doing less to do more is the concept behind Daily Practice #4 (Do The Thing), taking thirty minutes for yourself every single day will pay you back in energy, calmness, and joy. It won't always be easy—I wish it were—but I also promise it will 100 percent be worth it.

I wouldn't feel right sending you off without including a handy cheat sheet to skip to when you need a quick refresher, so you'll find it on the following pages.

Okay, are you ready to Do The Thing?

Let's get it done.

Love,
Andrea

CHEAT SHEET

## small moves, big life
### CHEAT SHEET

#### DAILY PRACTICE #1
#### BREATHE IN

**What you'll be doing:** breathwork to power up, slow down, and focus your intentions.

**When to do it:** mornings, first thing, and throughout the day.

**How long it will take:** 2 minutes.

#### DAILY PRACTICE #2
#### STRETCH YOURSELF

**What you'll be doing:** calming stretches to wake up your body, help prevent or mitigate chronic pain, and regulate your mood.

**When to do it:** mornings, right after breathwork.

**How long it will take:** 2 minutes.

CHEAT SHEET

### DAILY PRACTICE #3
### JUST PRESS PLAY

**What you'll be doing:** full-out effort, low-impact, 100 percent doable, sweaty, and fun mini-workouts.

**When to do it:** mornings, right after stretching.

**How long it will take:** 10 minutes.

### DAILY PRACTICE #4
### DO THE THING

**What you'll be doing:** achieving more by doing less via conscientious goal setting, upping your day-to-day productivity.

**When to do it:** mornings, right after your post-workout shower.

**How long it will take:** 2 minutes.

CHEAT SHEET

### DAILY PRACTICE #5
### SET THE TABLE

**What you'll be doing:** eating mindfully at breakfast (and eventually, every meal) and enjoying the unbeatable benefits of how you feel and function.

**When to do it:** mornings, right after your Do The Thing listmaking.

**How long it will take:** 10 minutes.

### DAILY PRACTICE #6
### MIND UP

**What you'll be doing:** using affirmations to learn to give yourself a break and love yourself, no matter how tough the going gets.

**When to do it:** mornings, right after breakfast or in the evening to set the stage for slumber.

**How long it will take:** 2 minutes.

CHEAT SHEET

DAILY PRACTICE #7
## BREATHE IT OUT

**What you'll be doing:** a no-nonsense, fail-safe bedtime routine so you can sleep with skill.

**When to do it:** evenings, right before you go to bed.

**How long it will take:** 2 minutes.

# acknowledgments

When my girls were little, I tried to teach them to make eye contact when thanking someone. "Now, look them in the eyes and say thank you," I would say. So many of us go through life mindlessly thanking our way through the day but very rarely connecting with the person on the other side of that gratitude—even if only for a few moments—so, I felt it was a valuable lesson to learn. As I write this final section of my book and close the chapter on one of my life's biggest dreams, I want to look some very special people in the eye and thank them properly for their contributions to this book.

Leigh and Laine, you are the greatest parts of me and the "thing" that makes me want to get up and Do The Thing every day. The pride I have in being your mother is like no other prize or accomplishment. You are a force of courage, kindness,

## ACKNOWLEDGMENTS

curiosity, and charisma (and you always make eye contact when you say thank you!). I am so grateful to watch you both grow into the amazing young women you are becoming. Continue to Sparkle & Shine in everything you do.

Winning the lottery isn't something I have often dreamed about (although I admit, that would be pretty damn cool). I have, however, always felt like I won the star prize being born the daughter of Debbie and John. Mom and Dad, your relentless support in making this tiny dancer run toward her very big dreams has become the foundation of my career and parenting. Knowing that I had you right behind me, guiding me, keeping my feet firmly on the ground, while reminding me that no dream was out of reach, is the reason I am the woman I am today. There are not enough "eye-to-eye thank-yous" to fully convey my gratitude.

It isn't often you meet someone in your professional life who instantly feels like a childhood friend, gabbing with them for hours and losing all track of time, but that is exactly what I found in Dan Jones. Dan, you made the challenges of writing this book one of the most enjoyable experiences. You brightened every hue, enhanced every memory, and brought my inner thoughts to life. Thank you for being such a wonderful teammate. Let's Do This Thing!

The journey to publishing this book started with a truly magical connection: meeting my agent, Todd Shuster. Thanks to him and his fantastic team: Jack Haug, Lauren Liebow, and

## ACKNOWLEDGMENTS

all at Aevitas Creative Management, past and present (hi, Daniella Cohen!).

A huge, heartfelt thanks to superstar editors Leah Wilson, Claire Schulz, and Stephanie Gorton, plus Kim Broderick, Morgan Carr, Anthony LaSasso, Glenn Yeffeth, and all at BenBella who believed in *Small Moves, Big Life* and gave it their trademark off-the-charts enthusiasm.

Finally, I want to take the time to thank the countless women in my life who have influenced this book and my personal journey. The women who entrusted me to guide, coach, and sculpt them into their happy, accomplished, Mind Up, confident selves—and who have taught me so many wonderful things along the way. You are the reason I love what I do, and I will forever be grateful for your faith and support.

# about the author

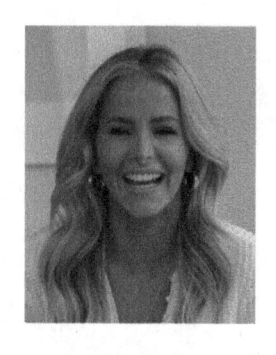

**Andrea Leigh Rogers** is a wellness entrepreneur, motivational coach, celebrity trainer, and creator of the groundbreaking fitness sensation Xtend Barre, a creative combination of traditional Pilates methods, ballet, and cardio. Featured in *Vogue*, *Harper's Bazaar*, and *Elle*, with live appearances on NBC, ABC, and CNN networks, she is a popular thought leader in health and movement communities and a youth skin care advocate; and her online workouts have been viewed millions of times.

Her lifelong love of movement started with a dedicated dance practice leading to a career as a professional dancer (most notably as principal dancer for Walt Disney World Co.), before mastering Pilates as a Comprehensive Classical trainer. Andrea then created her own innovative fusion of core, dance, and Pilates fundamentals, and encouraged by her clients' response, in 2008 she launched Xtend Barre, with locations worldwide.

A super trainer on US fitness streaming platform BODi since 2022, Andrea is also a motivational coach and speaker, focused on empowering women and girls, building community, and creating movement in all areas of life. She lives in Dallas, Texas, with her two daughters and their dog, Chedi.